BODY

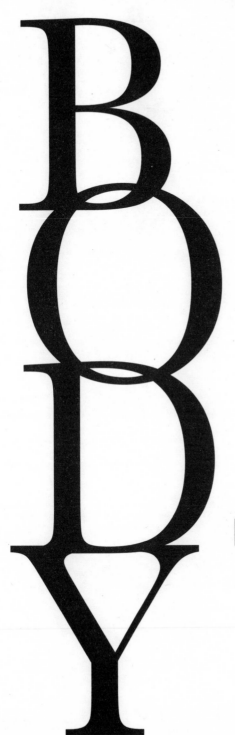

BODY

Simple techniques
and strategies to
**heal, reset
and restore**

JAMES
DAVIES

To my mum, my brothers

– the 'JET' team –

my wife, and my children

MEDICAL NOTE

This book contains advice and information relating to health care. It should be used to supplement rather than replace the advice of your doctor or another medical professional. If you know or suspect you have a health problem, it is recommended that you seek your physician's advice before embarking on any medical programme or treatment. All efforts have been made to ensure the accuracy of the information contained in this book as of the date of publication. This publisher and the author disclaim liability for any medical outcomes that may occur as a result of applying the methods suggested in this book. Additionally, some names and events have been changed to protect the privacy of the individuals involved. Occasionally, the author has shared treatment stories from his clients, whose consent has been sought for this purpose. Finally, some stories are hypothetical and appear purely for demonstration purposes.

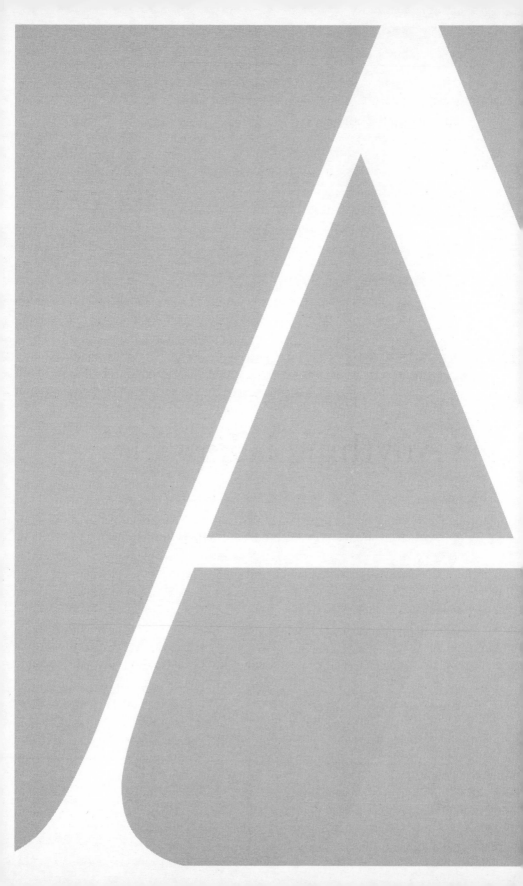

Anything is Possible

TALENT

When I was 12 years old, I had a plan. And it was a good one. I was going to represent Great Britain in the Olympics.

Now, before you dismiss me as some dreamer with his head in the clouds, at that time it was entirely possible. At 7 years old, I'd won my first school sport's day and knew I was the fastest in my class. From there, I quickly discovered that I was the fastest runner in my primary school; my friends and I would spend lunchtimes challenging everyone in the playground to see if they could beat me. No one could.

When I started secondary school, my PE teacher, Mr Raicevic, took me aside after football practice and told me I should start training properly, that I had real talent. He told me I was an all-rounder, but he thought I might have a future in running. To be singled out like that by my teacher propelled me forwards, made me think of the future and where I could be in a few years' time. Linford Christie was my idol; my nose had been pressed up against the TV screen when he won gold in Barcelona in 1992. To me, he was an example of what a normal person like me could achieve with talent and hard work. I was going to be the next Linford.

Running was my joy, my first love, and my passion. I found a freedom in it I had never experienced in a classroom. I'd struggled in school but not in the way that most people would imagine. It wasn't that I couldn't do the lessons or keep up with the work. It was more personal than that – I had a stammer. It could appear at any time, that familiar choking sensation. Sometimes I couldn't get my words out for what felt like minutes, my heart sinking whenever I was asked to read out loud in my English classes. A page of text seemed to take

DETER

a lifetime. I was never bullied, but some of my classmates did laugh. I tried not to be affected by it as I knew they weren't doing it cruelly. Therefore, to be told I was skilled at something I loved made me even more determined to prove myself.

At that young age I thought talent could get me anywhere. I trained hard and didn't mess around outside school. I was going to make it, I was sure of it – because I had talent, didn't I?

I was built for speed, excelled at short bursts in 100-metre and 200-metre races, but also enjoyed basketball, football, and even cross-country running. When I was around 13 years old, I started getting an ache in my lower back during the longer runs. I told myself it would be fine, couldn't conceive of there being anything wrong with the way

INVINCIBLE

I was training or treating my body. We did generic stretches at school, which I now know weren't suitable or effective. I ran off the aches and pains, or took a couple of days away from training, ignoring the dull throb until it went away. I was 13 years old. I was invincible.

All of this worked until, at 16 years old, my plan was left in tatters.

It was a cold autumnal day, the sort where you can see your breath in the crisp air, and I had been jogging on the spot. I was trying to keep my body warm as I waited for my turn to impress the PE examiner for one of my A-level assessments. Outside school I also trained with a local running club, had been winning district prizes for track and field, but didn't have the right coach or training routine.

When it was my turn to be assessed, I slid my feet against the blocks. My fingertips were splayed on the ground, my back ever so slightly rounded, hips directly aligned with my front toe, a position that I had practised so many times it felt like second nature. The examiner blew

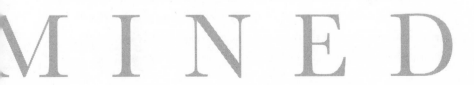

the whistle for me to start, and I was off, arms pumping. I knew I was doing well, was running really fast.

Ten strides in and a cramping sensation hit my thigh, just above my knee. I had never felt anything like it before – it was so strong that there was an accompanying electrical sensation. With the next step, I came crashing down and lay there for a moment, shock hardly registering as I was more concerned about being flat out on the ground in front of all my friends. When I pulled myself up and tried to run it off, I thought I was being sensible; it had worked in the past. My leg cramped again, and I knew that I would have to take a couple of days away from training. I limped over to the physiotherapist and he told me to apply heat, which I now know is the worst thing I could have done.

It all went downhill from there.

When a muscle is damaged and then poorly managed, the muscle tissue can sometimes calcify as if forming bone tissue. I eventually found out I had a condition called myositis ossificans, where this happens. No one realized this at the time. There was no attempt to diagnose what was wrong and instead, I went straight for treatment. First, I went to a massage therapist, who was aggressive in their treatment and made it worse. Then I saw a couple of physiotherapists who told me to exercise the muscle, and that damaged it as well. It sounds obvious, but if the correct diagnosis hasn't taken place, you might as well blindfold yourself

"I WAS ONLY 16 YEARS OLD AND WAS CERTAIN I WOULD GET BETTER."

and point randomly at a chart when deciding on a course of treatment. Some might help, some might hinder.

Eventually I had an MRI scan, which showed I had a muscle tear that had turned into calcified tissue. I had two options: a steroid injection, or an operation. After some consideration I went with surgery, which was the worst decision I have ever made. I lost a large part of the muscle and there wasn't the aftercare that I needed. Every time I tensed the muscle, I could see that part of it was missing.

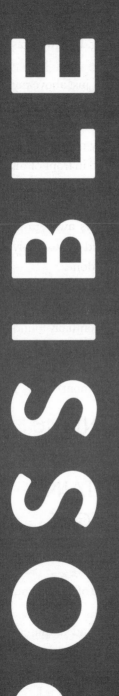

POSSIBLE

But I still had hope. I was only 16 years old and was certain I would get better. My family and friends were always telling people I was going to be in the Olympics. 'James is going to make it. You'll see him on TV soon, better ask for his autograph now while you know him!' I used to smile at the attention, joke along with them, hoping that I would prove them right.

Weeks turned into months and I began trying out for the Great Britain team, injured but still showing up every day. It was the first time I lost races. At 17 years old, no one was talking about my future any more.

When the Great Britain team started accepting into its ranks people I used to win races against, but not me, I reluctantly gave up on the dream that had carried me through my teenage years. I had learnt that talent can only get you so far. To really succeed you need the right training methods, coaches, and therapists supporting you.

So, there I was – 17 years old, no plan, dodgy leg, and no idea of who I was any more. Not the greatest starting point for a young man who had thought he could achieve anything he wanted with hard work and talent. If I'm honest, it was a pretty dark time. My parents had recently separated, and it was just me and my mum living together as my older brothers had left for university. It was a very loving family, but I felt that I had to hold everything inside and just keep going. It wasn't long before I realized that I needed a new plan.

I knew that I wasn't meant for a desk job, and that I would struggle with anything that required me to talk all day because of my stammer. I still thought about the Olympics constantly, even more now that it was beyond my grasp. But then I started thinking about it differently, looking at it from another angle: I might not be able to run in the Olympics, but I could still help other athletes achieve their dream. One thing I was certain of was that I didn't want anyone else to go through what I had experienced. I set a new long-term goal: I would work with track and field athletes in Team GB as an official therapist.

I began researching how I could help people, what type of therapy complemented my skills. I soon narrowed it down to doctor, osteopath, or physiotherapist, but it wasn't until I started looking seriously into osteopathy that I knew I had found my calling. Osteopaths use their hands to diagnose and are trained for four years in anatomy as well as neuroscience, pharmacology and pathology. Osteopathy has been a recognized practice for over a hundred years, and osteopaths use methods of manual therapy to alleviate and prevent injuries and general deterioration. More importantly, they look at the body as a whole, understanding that everything is connected, rather than focusing specifically on the spine, soft tissues, or nervous system. It was this holistic approach that convinced me it was the right choice.

"I WAS NOW AN 18-YEAR-OLD WITH A PLAN."

I was now an 18-year-old with a plan.

Four years of university passed quickly as I immersed myself in learning about the human body. I still had my stammer, still feared having to give presentations to the class, but I persevered, despite a small part of me worrying that people would think I was unintelligent because I struggled to articulate my thoughts. I also learnt more about my own injury through my studies, that there had been early warning signs because of the pain in my lower back. I began to appreciate how different parts of the body work in unison, and that a warning flag in one area could mean a devastating injury in another.

Once I had qualified, I was able to immediately start working – another reason I had chosen this career path. My parents had brought me up to work ten times harder than anyone else, so I threw myself into setting up my practice. I wanted to work with everyone I could and help eradicate their pain, from 90-year-olds to women in their third trimester of pregnancy. Looking back, I don't know how I sustained those fourteen-hour days, but it was where I learnt my craft. Alongside all of this, I also treated young athletes, who were at the critical period of turning professional, providing them with the help that could save them from the type of career-ending injury I had experienced.

Unsurprisingly, I still had my eye on the Olympics. At the time that I qualified it was unheard of for an osteopath to work in sports, which had traditionally been the domain of physiotherapists. I was going against the tide by pushing to work with athletes, but I did it anyway. I started treating some of the junior GB Team athletes in my private practice, which led to me treating the senior ones as well. Through word of mouth, I was also recommended to American and Caribbean athletes when they visited the UK for competitions.

My results were getting me noticed and I was invited to join British Athletics. But there was a catch – and it was a big one. I'd have to close my practice for four years, just for the chance of being picked for the Olympics team of therapists. It was a huge risk, but I took it, determined to achieve my dream. I threw myself into improving the athletes' performance, healing their injuries, and trying to prevent further ones from happening.

And then I got the call I'd been waiting years for. I was asked by the Great Britain team to join them as a therapist for the Rio Olympics in 2016, to treat the athletes that I used to win races against when I was 16 years old. My mind was only just beginning to understand that all the risks, all the sacrifices, strain, work, compromises, and pressures had been worth it.

I'd done it.

MISSION ACCOMPLISHED.

I was 30 years old and had achieved my absolute dream. So, why wasn't I completely happy with my life?

On the flight back to the UK from Rio I took the time to consider my life and where I was. I had two young children and a wife who I loved very much. If I continued to chase international work and the Olympics, then I would miss out on those precious years when my children were shaped into the adults they would become. It was also around this time that my dad sadly passed away. He was a civil engineer living in India and a classic workaholic. Work was all he focused on and there was no balance to his life. Consequently, he had neglected himself and paid the ultimate price.

"I WAS 30 AND HAD ACHIEVED MY ABSOLUTE DREAM. SO WHY WASN'T I COMPLETELY HAPPY WITH MY LIFE?"

I knew I had to learn from what had happened to him and find some balance. I still had more to achieve, but I knew I had to be smarter about how I worked. So, I took my sights off the international scene and looked at what I could do in the UK. I set up my practice again and word spread.

My ethos has always been, *Anything is possible.* That is my baseline. Instead of telling someone who has injured themselves running that they can never run again, I work with the client to explore methods that will have them lacing up their trainers again and heading outside for a run. I've worked with so many people who have been told by therapists that they will never again do the hobby they love. This is something I strongly disagree with – it's taking the easy route. Instead

PERFORMA

> **"IF I COULD EXPLAIN TO PEOPLE WHY THEY HAVE PAIN, THEY COULD PLAY A MORE ACTIVE ROLE IN THEIR TREATMENT."**

of saying 'no', I want to explore whether it's possible. There's so much joy in those clients when they are told they can still try.

Soon I was treating Premiership footballers, and film stars, and those who might not be household names but whose ailments were just as important to me, such as the fireman who came to me with lower-back pain which I realized was possibly prostate cancer, and which was then caught in the early stages. Over the years I was lucky enough to treat people such as David Beckham, Kylie Minogue, and Eva Mendes, to name just a few. Who would have thought, when I was a 10-year-old watching David Beckham scoring from the halfway line, that one day I would treat him?

One highlight of my career was treating my hero, Linford Christie, when the Great Britain team was training in Cape Town. When he walked into the room we would share for six weeks, I suddenly turned back into that 7-year-old boy, who had realized for the first time that anything was possible.

Since the Rio Olympics, I'd started taking on clients as a performance coach, helping them achieve their dreams, ranging from completing their first marathon all the way to joining a particular rugby union team. I found the right coaches, trainers, and therapists for them. It was a full package deal, a 360-degree road map. I'd mentor them and build the best team so they could achieve their goals. My diary was packed, and I knew that if I treated ten people a day the quality of

NCE COACH

that treatment would inevitably drop. I was only one person, with two hands. How could I help more people?

I knew then that I had to write a book. If I could explain to people why they have pain, teach them how to be involved in their diagnosis, and advise on the different therapies available, they could play a more active role in their treatment. I researched the market and there was nothing else like it.

I also want people to be more aware of how their bodies function and that small steps, such as moving our bodies throughout the day, can lead to huge benefits. The body is such a unique and precious thing, and we need to take care of it. Sometimes we forget that. It's also a complex system and needs to be treated with respect. Everyone assumes that as we get older, our movement decreases significantly, but that isn't true. There are ways to limit this. I've been very fortunate through my work to travel the world and see other ways of living, which has shaped my way of thinking. Some people I met may not have had much money, but they were healthy and could hold a squatting position for hours. I would watch in awe as people in their eighties nimbly leaned down and touched their toes. How many of us can do that?

"YOU DON'T HAVE TO BE SKINNY OR RIPPED TO BE HEALTHY."

But change is possible. *Anything is possible.* And you don't need to set aside hours of your day to achieve it – I know that isn't realistic for most of us. Instead, I've learnt over the years that the best way of incorporating change is to fit it into your daily routine. I did it with my own stammer: I was too busy for hours of therapy each week, so practised breathing techniques as I got dressed in the morning.

Also, I don't believe in focusing only on losing weight or gaining muscle. The message we often hear is that to be healthy you must lose weight. Of course, there is an element of truth to that when people are significantly overweight. But I want to be clear that you don't have to be skinny or ripped to be healthy. What matters is what's going on inside. Whatever your shape, if you can't fully express yourself through movement then that is something that needs correcting, and I can show you how.

Over the last ten years my stammer has turned from what is classed as an 'overt' one to a 'covert' one. Nowadays, most people I meet don't realize I have a stammer, but that doesn't mean it has gone away. It's still always there, lurking beneath the surface, and I have to constantly control it, which can be exhausting. It will catch up with me on a day when I'm overtired or stressed, usually with such bad timing that I have to smile. I'll never be free of it, but I've gone from having a stammer to being someone who makes others feel at ease when I talk to them. People confide in me, ask me for advice. I've turned what I thought was my weakness into a strength. And on the bad days, when my stammer interferes in my life, I can help people through my writing, when the words flow and are fixed to the page.

"I'VE TURNED WHAT I THOUGHT WAS MY WEAKNESS INTO A STRENGTH."

It's one of the many gratifying examples that 'anything is possible' with the right methods in place.

ANYTHING IS POSSIBLE

HOW TO USE THE BOOK

Anyone who has spent a lot of time with me knows that I love to plan and problem-solve. Through hard work, I achieved all the things I set out to do, such as working at the Olympics, treating Premiership football players and American football NFL players, and prepping actors for movie roles. Most importantly, I learnt how to treat my clients in the most effective way to help reduce their pain and move forwards with their lives.

I was successful, busy, flying somewhere every week, and I knew I was fortunate to travel around the world. But something wasn't right. Every year, around the same time when I was in Norway with my family, having the closest thing I ever got to a holiday, I would always get ill either with an upset stomach or vomiting. It always happened after a long season of track and field or football. When it was time to rest, my body would collapse as I was no longer running on adrenaline. It took a few years, but I eventually realized that I didn't have any balance in my life.

I needed to problem-solve *me*.

This is what led to me taking a step backwards, mapping out what was important in my life: me time, family time, and working smarter instead of harder. This self-reflection made me realize that I was not alone in having little balance in my life. For the past fifteen years I have seen the same pattern in my patients who are always rushing around on full throttle. They would tell me:

'I don't have time.'

'I'll take a break when I go on holiday next year.'

'I'll relax when I retire.'

I would give them all my best advice, but I wasn't practising it myself. So, I started to take ice baths, saunas, and jacuzzis every day, and I devised the road map that I'm about to share with you. For the first time I started to put myself first and, in doing that, everything in my life slotted into place.

This book was written to fit in with your busy lifestyle. Instead of adding another chore or unwanted commitment to your life, it will be an aid and point of reference that can be immediately accessed and understood. People learn in different ways, so there are lots of illustrations, text boxes with more in-depth information, and symbols to signify the core facts you will need. Here are the main ones you need to know about:

These are the warning flags we should all be aware of, as they indicate a more serious condition that might require immediate medical attention.

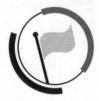

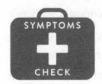

The symptoms checks are a general tool that help you decide if there is a potential condition that needs exploring. We use these to test our body for levels of pain or restrictions in movement.

This is a quick-fire self-diagnosis test for a specific condition.

These help diagnose a specific condition with a step-by-step guide.

These are the treatments that will help you recover from each injury or condition. They are split into ones you can do at home and others that you might need professional help with from a therapist.

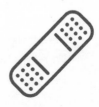

I've always hoped that after reading this book it will find a place on an easily reached shelf in your home, brought down every time a friend or relative pops around and mentions a new pain they've been feeling in their shoulder or hip. Together you can then turn to the right section and begin your diagnosis. So that it can become the reference book you will use for years, it has been broken down into four sections:

PART ONE

KNOWLEDGE IS POWER

This is an overview of pain. It lays the foundations we all need to understand the messages our bodies are sending. Here we are introduced to the tools we will use to assess and describe our pain so we can then diagnose the condition behind it.

PART TWO

PARTS OF THE BODY:
DIAGNOSIS AND TREATMENT

In this part, the body has been sectioned off into eleven distinct areas so you can jump straight into whatever interests you. The idea with these chapters is that you read about the areas in which you have experienced pain, or have an interest in, and then move on to the third part about working with a therapist and treatments. Or, you might decide to read through them all. It's completely up to you.

BODY

BODY

THERAPISTS AND THERAPIES

This is where we start thinking about what treatments we might need and who is best placed to provide them. Have you ever wondered what exactly clicking or cupping is and when it should be used? Or what the difference is between a physiotherapist and a chiropractor? This is where you will find out.

PART FOUR

RESET AND BODY FREEDOM

These are some simple steps you can take to keep your body in peak condition and enjoy that freedom of movement we all need to live pain-free. Because prevention is always better than a cure, I've laid out the small adjustments you can make in a road map that is easy to understand and slots right into your life.

Finally, there is a helpful list of key terms for you to read through and refer back to, as we won't be explaining these terms every time they come up in the text (or the book would be twice as long). This means we can move on to describing, diagnosing, treating and preventing your pain in the quickest, most direct way... all leading to you problem-solving your own conditions and ultimately gaining balance in your own life.

KEY TERMS

Acupuncture: A treatment in which a needle is inserted into the skin to try and balance the flow of *qi*. It is used for pain relief, general ailments, or to target specific problems such as addiction to cigarettes.

Chiropractor: A therapist who specializes in the nervous system and the diagnosis and treatment of disorders involving the muscles and nerves. They are known for treating neck and back conditions, but can cover all areas of the body. Their treatment predominantly involves mobilization or clicking (i.e. manipulation) of the joints, as well as massage.

Clicking: A treatment that is used when there is a restriction of movement in a joint. A therapist will use a short thrust to 'click' to restore the normal function and movement of the joint. It is also known as manipulation, cracking, or high-velocity thrusts.

Cold laser therapy: A treatment that uses low-level laser light to stimulate tissue repair and circulation.

Colonic:	Colonic irrigation, or colonic hydrotherapy, is the practice of inserting a tube into the rectum and then pumping warm water into the colon. The water is then drained back out bringing all the waste products in your bowel with it.
Cupping:	The therapeutic practice of placing a cup onto the skin, which creates a vacuum. The suction from the cup improves circulation and draws the blood to the surface of the skin.
Dry needling:	A treatment that is also known as 'medical acupuncture' and considered the 'Western' version of acupuncture. A fine needle is inserted under the skin, which provides a stimulus that sends a signal to the brain that there has been an injury to the area. The brain responds by increasing blood flow to the area. It is effective in reducing sensitivity in areas where the muscle is tight.
Osteopath:	A therapist who treats the body's structures through massage, mobilization, and clicking (manipulation) of the joints, as well as encouraging the circulation of blood throughout the body to all the tissues. Osteopaths believe in treating the body as a whole and therefore the skeleton, muscles, ligaments, and connective tissues must work well together.

Performance therapy:	A form of therapy that aims to improve the mechanics and function of a patient to perform a skill, activity, or event. This is usually a quick, effective session of therapy performed by a highly skilled therapist.
Physiotherapist:	A therapist who takes a 'whole-person' approach to a patient and aims to restore function and movement to the body through exercises, massaging the tissues, as well as via mobilization and manipulation of the joints. Patients are often provided with exercises to continue at home.
Pilates:	A form of exercise that aims to strengthen the body, with a particular emphasis on posture, balance, flexibility, and core strength.
Podiatrist:	Previously known as a 'chiropodist'. Podiatry is a branch of medicine that deals with conditions and disorders of the feet and ankles. Podiatrists can perform surgery on ingrown toenails, as well as deal with common conditions such as verrucas, corns, fungal infections, and feet that are affected by diabetes.

Surface anatomy:	The study of the outside of the body, without the need for dissection, to learn where the internal structures are.
Tecar therapy:	A treatment that uses an electrical current to reduce pain and inflammation, and to decrease healing time.
TENS machine:	A transcutaneous electrical nerve stimulation (TENS) machine that offers a method of pain relief involving the use of a mild electrical current. Helps the recovery from a traumatic injury or if a person is training very hard for a sporting event.
Traction:	Pulling on one aspect of a joint to create a separation of the surfaces that meet to make a joint.
Ultrasound:	A treatment that uses sound waves to help with circulation, reducing pain, and increasing the rate of healing. The sound waves can also produce images of the inside of the body to help diagnose a condition.
Yoga:	A form of exercise that involves holding poses that aid flexibility while concentrating on your breathing. It can help with meditation as well.

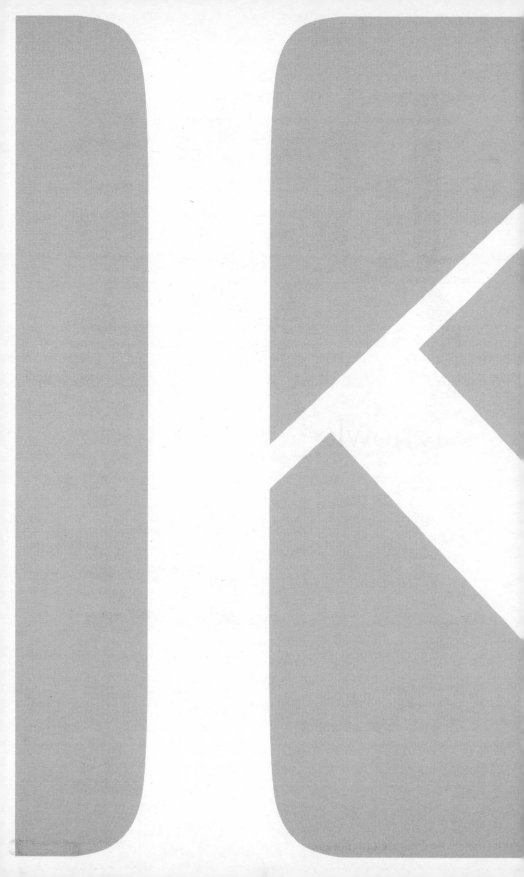

PART ONE:

Knowledge Is Power

CHAPTER 1:

Origins
of Pain

Whenever we feel pain, it is a message from our body that something isn't quite right and it needs our attention. Often, we ignore it and carry on as before. Sometimes we try to treat it, but it doesn't get any better.

We haven't realized that we have missed out a crucial step: diagnosis. Without the correct diagnosis, we cannot expect the right treatment, and this is where I want to help you become your own pain detective.

From our earliest ancestors, the feeling of pain has been our first alert system that something is wrong – that we shouldn't press down harder on that sharp rock, or we should take our hand away from the fire. It is a neural system set to protect our bodies from further damage, urging us to look after ourselves and try to heal. We've been taught that pain is wrong, evil even; but in its simplest form, it can be a lifesaver.

But what about the subtler types of pain? The ones that creep up on us, which we are too busy to attend to. The ones we ignore in the hope they will go away. They are just as important, as they are the first warning signs that more, and often worse, is to come. Pain is something we often live in fear of, yet we don't always take all the steps we can to prevent it.

Then there is the other end of the spectrum – the continuous chronic pain that we might not know the source of. It can affect every

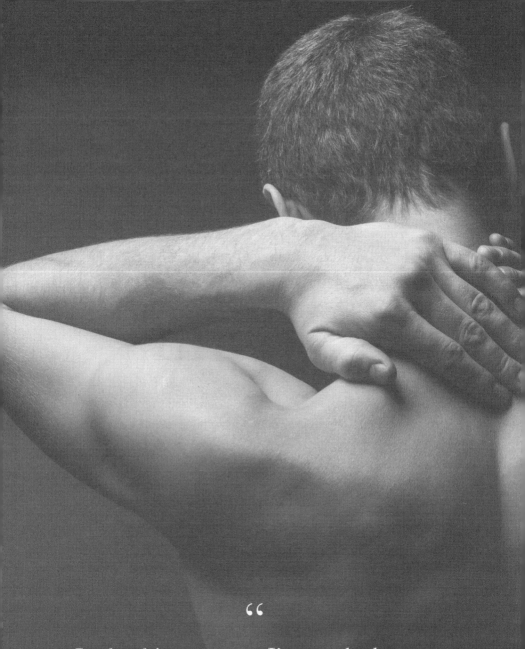

"

In the thirteen years I've worked as an osteopath I have seen every type of pain.

"

area of our lives, interfere with our sleep, take away our pleasure in the activities that used to bring us joy, as well as affect our mental and emotional wellbeing. When we can't decipher what our bodies are telling us, then we can't begin to heal.

In the thirteen years I've worked as an osteopath I have seen every conceivable type and spectrum of pain. They are all messages from our bodies telling us that something is wrong, something needs to be adjusted or healed. The difficulty is finding the source. Once there is a correct diagnosis, then the right treatment can be put in place.

"I BEGAN TO THINK ABOUT HOW THE PATIENT COULD HELP."

But the correct diagnosis can take time. A multitude of information needs to be filtered and sorted. Time is often something that our medical professionals are not given. Cuts to the NHS and staffing levels have left them with no choice but to do the best they can in a limited window. This is something I often see when I meet patients who have spent years trying to find out the root cause of their condition.

This was why I began to think about how the patient could help. As an osteopath I spent four years studying anatomy and learning the difference between a healthy and unhealthy muscle just by touch. But no one understands a patient's own body as intimately as they do. What they don't know is the right questions to ask themselves and the diagnoses those answers will lead to. They can spend hours googling symptoms on the internet, coming out with one potential diagnosis after another, some so extreme that they slam their laptop shut and are scared to open it again for a few days. Understandably, they push the problem away and it lingers there until they can face it again. Or it comes back, more aggressively this time, and they are forced to seek help.

I wanted to find a way that the patient could help with their diagnosis and then take steps to find the right treatment. I want to solve the case of *you* by exploring every aspect of your life and the various treatments that are available for *your* condition. The last thing I want is someone spending their hard-earned money on something that won't help. Later on, I'll also talk about what you can do at home to help your recovery for all budgets and lifestyles.

Then, once you are living pain-free, you'll want to keep it that way and there are many small adjustments you can make to keep your body nimble and supple. As we all know, prevention is better than cure.

As tempting as it is to jump straight into diagnosis, we need to first know what we are dealing with – we wouldn't try and learn the piano without listening to music beforehand. As naturally fearful as we are of pain, I hope that by understanding it and having a firm grasp of why it exists, I can curb some of its perplexity and reduce it to something that is controllable, that we can contemplate tackling, managing, and often defeating.

DESCRIBING PAIN

Sharp, hot, electrical, dull, aching, debilitating ... these are just some of the many ways to describe it, but what is pain? Put in the simplest way, the brain is our main control system and pain is a message. Pain is a communication between the nervous system and spinal cord telling the brain that something is wrong. The brain then processes that information, and the pain is perceived.

FIG. 1.1 THE FOUR MAIN TYPES ARE:

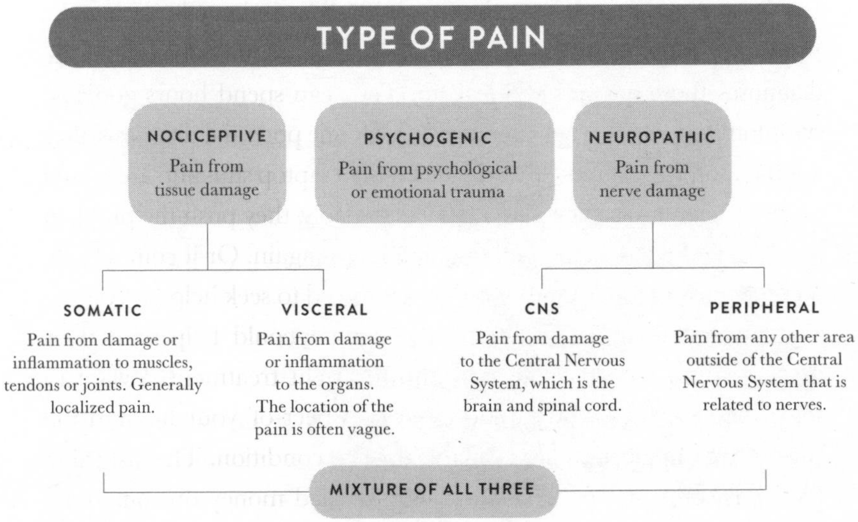

TYPE OF PAIN

NOCICEPTIVE	PSYCHOGENIC	NEUROPATHIC
Pain from tissue damage	Pain from psychological or emotional trauma	Pain from nerve damage

SOMATIC	VISCERAL	CNS	PERIPHERAL
Pain from damage or inflammation to muscles, tendons or joints. Generally localized pain.	Pain from damage or inflammation to the organs. The location of the pain is often vague.	Pain from damage to the Central Nervous System, which is the brain and spinal cord.	Pain from any other area outside of the Central Nervous System that is related to nerves.

MIXTURE OF ALL THREE

NOCICEPTIVE PAIN:

This is pain caused by soft tissue damage such as the torn muscle I had at 16 years old. Typically, this is caused by an injury, illness, or disease. Types of nociceptive are fractures, sprains, irritable bowel syndrome (IBS), and gastritis. These pains are often described as sharp, aching, throbbing, or a pinprick sensation.

PSYCHOGENIC PAIN:

This is pain from psychological or emotional trauma that is a real feeling of pain, but with no physical trauma.

NEUROPATHIC PAIN:

This is pain from nerve damage or irritation. Types I see regularly in my practice are a disc bulge pressing on a nerve, or a trapped nerve in the neck. These pains are often described as tingling, burning, shooting, or sensitive to touch.

MIXTURE OF ALL THREE:

Often you can be left battling pain from a combination of the above. Common examples of this are fibromyalgia, cancer, or post-surgery pain.

There are many ways to classify pain, but I like to break it down into four categories (see Figure 1.1).

This is a textbook answer and a good starting point. But I believe in describing each *individual's* pain. If I want to describe *your* pain, then the first thing I need is a pain scale. Not so I can add a pretty diagram, or because I believe that you've never considered rating your pain on a 0–10 basis before. It's because we all need to be on the same page. One person's debilitation is another's niggle, and that's absolutely fine. This isn't about judgement or fortitude. It's about making sure we all rate our pain in the same way, so we can decide when you need medical attention and, later on, whether you can exercise throughout your recovery.

It's also so that you can explain to medical professionals the intensity of what you are feeling. How many times have we been to the doctor and tried to explain our pain, or what is wrong, and ended up mumbling, 'I mean, it can get bad, sometimes really bad, and then other times it's a bit better, you know?' Wouldn't it be much clearer if we could bring our own pain scale to the appointment, that we've considered beforehand, rather than being expected to give a snap answer? If that were the case, we could sit down and say, 'If I've slept well, it's a three in the morning, levelling up to a five if I've been load-bearing all day, sometimes nudging into a six if I've twisted it or picked up something really heavy.'

Below is the pain scale I've created (see Figure 1.2), and it is the first tool for what I like to call a 'Symptoms Check', which will help you diagnose your pain. Thankfully, most people won't experience a level nine or ten in their lifetime, but we still need to cover every level of pain.

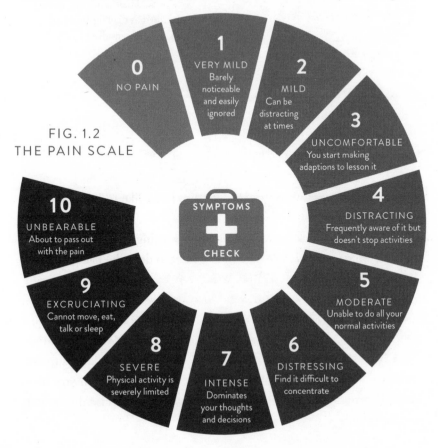

FIG. 1.2
THE PAIN SCALE

0 NO PAIN

1 VERY MILD
Barely noticeable and easily ignored

2 MILD
Can be distracting at times

3 UNCOMFORTABLE
You start making adaptions to lesson it

4 DISTRACTING
Frequently aware of it but doesn't stop activities

5 MODERATE
Unable to do all your normal activities

6 DISTRESSING
Find it difficult to concentrate

7 INTENSE
Dominates your thoughts and decisions

8 SEVERE
Physical activity is severely limited

9 EXCRUCIATING
Cannot move, eat, talk or sleep

10 UNBEARABLE
About to pass out with the pain

SYMPTOMS
CHECK

The highest I've ever reached is a level eight, when I slammed the boot of my car on my hand. As I'm sure you can imagine, the initial pain was so bad I actually cried (even thinking about it now makes me shudder), but the resulting nerve damage kept me at an eight, as I couldn't sleep or do much with that arm.

When rating your pain, always rate it at its peak. If the pain is a one or two then it's usually something that you should just keep a close eye on without needing further investigation. It's likely it's not a serious issue unless you have felt the pain for a few months. If it lasts for more than a couple of months, then it needs your attention. However, as with all things, trust your instincts. If you think it needs medical attention now, then you should see a doctor. Better safe than sorry.

When I tore my quad muscle at 16 years old, I would rate my pain as a level five and it therefore needed immediate medical attention. The backache I started getting at 13 years old was a level three. My body was trying to tell me that it needed attention and I ignored it.

> "WHEN I TORE MY QUAD MUSCLE AT 16 YEARS OLD, I WOULD RATE MY PAIN AS A LEVEL FIVE."

When you're nudging into a level three and you start making *adaptations* to lessen it, you need to do something about your pain. This is because you will ask other areas of your body to compensate: for example, you can't use your right hand much, so you expect your left to take the strain without building up to it; or you find it painful to press down on the ball of your foot, so you push your hip out and put more weight on the other leg. Once you start making changes to your posture, gait, lifestyle, or in my case, running technique, then the pain needs investigating. Every adjustment you make can cause later damage to another part of your body. Even if you have been doing this for years, it's better to try and reduce or reverse the damage now rather than ignoring it.

So, the first step to describing pain is to give it a number. But that's not enough. We also need to describe the *character* of our pain. We need to flesh it out, give it several layers, because different types of pain indicate different problems.

Now I know memory aids aren't everyone's cup of tea, but this is one I use to ensure all aspects of pain's character are covered. If we can describe pain in a rounded way, we will know whether it is a pain that requires immediate attention. It also makes it easier when describing it to medical professionals and frees up their time so they can advise or treat you.

I use the following questions (STOP) to help people describe their pain.

USING THE MNEMONIC STOP TO DESCRIBE PAIN:

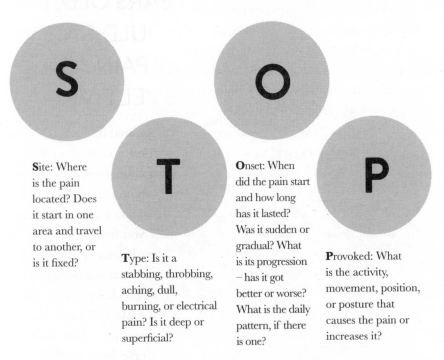

Site: Where is the pain located? Does it start in one area and travel to another, or is it fixed?

Type: Is it a stabbing, throbbing, aching, dull, burning, or electrical pain? Is it deep or superficial?

Onset: When did the pain start and how long has it lasted? Was it sudden or gradual? What is its progression – has it got better or worse? What is the daily pattern, if there is one?

Provoked: What is the activity, movement, position, or posture that causes the pain or increases it?

The **S**ite of the pain can help narrow down the location of an injury. It also provides a clue as to whether it is nerve or tissue pain, because if it's a pain that travels, it's more likely to be nerve pain. The **T**ype of pain is so important. If it's a sharp or stabbing pain, then this is a sign of a more serious problem that needs your immediate attention. Words like 'burning', 'electrical', or 'tingling' indicate nerve pain, whereas 'sharp', 'dull', or 'aching' are more likely to be tissue damage. **O**nset is equally important, as we'll see later, because even a level one pain that you've had for several months needs your attention. How the pain is **P**rovoked can help diagnose the **T**ype of tissue or nerve pain you have.

If you're in pain now or have felt pain recently, give it a number from the pain scale and try to assess it using STOP. And remember that when rating your pain, you should always rate it at its peak. It's important to use these two together and get into the habit of using them whenever you feel a new pain.

You now have your first tools for diagnosing pain.

> **"YOU NOW HAVE YOUR FIRST TOOLS FOR DIAGNOSING PAIN."**

PAIN FROM INACTIVITY

We often think of pain as coming from an action – we've stood on a nail, or whacked our elbow against the wall. But when it comes to pain, it's just as important to think about what you *haven't* done. As human beings we are meant to be active. We are designed as foragers, so our bodies expect to walk around for six hours a day, occasionally expelling huge amounts of energy as we sprint away from a tiger.

Instead, we live in an era when we get up in the morning and drive or take public transport. We sit in the same place for eight hours, escaping briefly to buy a sandwich if we have time. We then get back in our car and drive home, sitting clogged up in traffic jams and feeling exhausted.

We've all been tired after a long drive or a particularly stressful day. We've exhausted ourselves, but when you stop to think about it, we haven't actually *moved*. We're tired from having to concentrate the entire time, not from physical exertion.

Pain from inactivity has become increasingly prevalent in the last fifty years and has expanded further following the Covid-19 pandemic. We all know this. The combination of people losing their daily commute and the chance to walk a few kilometres has been replaced with long working hours at unstable makeshift desks. There have been huge surges in neck pain and lower-back pain because of poor posture and inactivity. People who were regular gym-goers stopped their usual routines and that led to them to being injured when they were able to restart.

"PAIN FROM INACTIVITY HAS BECOME PREVALENT IN THE LAST FIFTY YEARS."

Our bodies are designed to be used and they're designed to be tested. We have to get everything pumping on a daily basis as this affects our circulation and regulates the body. The fact that we need to go to the gym means we're not doing enough during the day. Most of us know we don't move enough so when we do get to the gym, we punish ourselves and try and fit in the six hours of walking we're missing into one or two hours. If you think about it, we're sprinting away from tigers for two hours, rather than doing the gentler exercise our bodies need as well.

A few small changes can make a huge difference, and I'll take you through the most beneficial ones later on. Even a few stretches before sitting down can help alleviate those daily niggles and aches that so many people suffer from. Or you can do stretches in the car for your neck and shoulders. We need that fun freedom of movement back in our lives and not be scared of looking stupid on the motorway when we're rolling our shoulders in a traffic jam. We should also incorporate these things into our lives when we are pain-free, because why wait to feel pain when you can prevent it instead?

ACUTE PAIN IS
TEMPORARY

CHRONIC PAIN

The chances are that at some point you have suffered from chronic pain. The term 'chronic' can make us think of people who find it difficult to function because of permanent, debilitating pain. But this isn't exactly right; it's much more encompassing because chronic pain doesn't have to be constant. It can come and go during the day, but many people don't realize that when a pain leaves us for weeks, months, or even years, it will still be classified as *chronic* pain if it returns, as long as it's in the same site and is the same type of pain. If it recurs, then it's chronic pain. So, welcome to the Chronic Pain Club! I'm already a member because of an ongoing shoulder injury that I'm currently treating, so let me show you around.

As you've already seen, there are different ways to sort and classify pain, but medical professionals usually start with either 'acute' or 'chronic'. *Acute* pain is temporary, such as a sprained ankle or a second-degree burn. You pay your dues, your body heals, and you move on, perhaps a little more wary of lunging for that basketball or juggling cooking dinner with making a cup of coffee, but you are nevertheless healed and pain-free.

Chronic pain is ongoing, usually for a period of more than three to six months. It doesn't describe the severity of the pain, but instead refers to the time it is experienced. You can have the most searing momentary pain, but it will still be classed as acute. Instead, it will be a continuous dull ache that someone else lives with for months that will be classified as chronic pain.

Chronic pain also doesn't have to be debilitating. In fact, it's often a level three on the pain scale, so we can get away with ignoring it. There will be trails of pain and we might not realize we have chronic pain, so we make a few small adaptations and carry on. With these low levels of pain, you should think of your body as a friend, knocking on your door, saying, 'Sorry to bother you, but I'm letting you know that something isn't quite right. What's that? You're really busy and can't deal with it right now? Oh, well, I'll come back soon and try again.' It tries a few more times over the next few months, but you're still too busy. A year later, it's back, but it's not knocking on your door any more. Instead, it's blown the door right off its hinges and you're left wondering how this happened. Pain has all your attention now.

But while it's still trying to get your attention, other things are happening inside your body that you might not be aware of. The body is clever in that it learns to adapt to pain, and we need to realize that those long-term adaptions aren't always the best thing for us. It all goes back to our pain scale: level three is when you need to ask, 'Am I making adaptations to lessen the pain?' Level two and even level one need attention if the pain has been there for over three months.

"THE BODY IS CLEVER IN THAT IT LEARNS TO ADAPT TO PAIN."

People think pain is part of getting older, that they should be feeling aches. But it's not. The knee joint is a classic example of this. We all assume that as we get older our knees will give in, that it's a natural deterioration, but the knee pain we're feeling can be because the joint is slightly out of sync. When you straighten your leg there is a screw-home mechanism in your knee for the last fifteen degrees, and if it gets stuck, it causes wear and tear. People live with this for years, then play a friendly game of football one day and tear their cruciate ligament.

CHRONIC PAIN IS ONGOING

THREE OF THE WORST PAINS

1. **TRIGEMINAL NEURALGIA:**
   This is a sudden sharp shooting pain through the cranial nerve in the jaw that lasts for a few seconds, but can happen several times a day. A client once told me that they would rather chew glass than experience that pain again.

   ....

2. **PHANTOM LIMB PAIN:**
   This is when someone feels pain in an amputated limb that is no longer there. Originally, doctors thought it was a type of psychological pain, but now they believe it is damaged nerve endings, or the nerves actually 'rewiring'.

   ....

3. **SLIPPED DISC THAT PRESSES ON THE NERVES:**
   This is when the tissue between the bones in your spine moves and presses on the nerves. Patients with this condition usually can't get out of bed for the first few days, or even weeks, of their recovery.

Chronic pain doesn't always serve an obvious 'purpose'. You hit your thumb with a hammer and your thumb tells you straightaway not to do that again. Instead, chronic pain can occur when there is no obvious injury, disease, or illness that has caused it. The shift from your medical practitioners might start to turn from diagnosis to 'management'. Management of pain is crucial and there will be more on that later in the book. Alternatively, there may be a clear reason for your chronic pain, which no longer serves a purpose, but it just keeps on going. You've heard the smoke alarm and are attending to the burnt potatoes in the oven, but it just keeps on beeping, even though you've pressed the reset button multiple times and removed its batteries – the smoke alarm is plugged into the mains and there is no way of appeasing it.

As a society, we often treat the symptoms rather than the source. People get stuck in a loop of painkillers and steroid injections for a couple of months of relief and then they're back to square one again. Eventually the doctors can't give them any more injections as their guidelines say that after three or four, the patient should have surgery. They're now on track for an operation, because they can no longer have steroid injections, and their treatment plans are accelerating out of their control as the months and years pass.

Most of my patients come to me after they've exhausted all the possibilities, seen different types of medical professionals, but still don't have any answers. They're running out of ideas. I love treating chronic pain because it forces me to look at the finer details – every aspect of the patient's life – and this is how we are going to approach your pain as well. We need to look at the individual rather than give a textbook answer. Chronic pain is all about the bigger picture rather than taking a reductionist viewpoint.

In my practice, I go right back to when the patient first felt the pain and explore how it came about. This is the same method we will use here with STOP. I ask: What were they doing at the time? Did it come on suddenly or was it gradual? It also helps to explore the different types of treatment they've had in the past and whether they worked. I also look at their diagnosis. Many people have been told what the issue is, but sometimes it's incorrect. Instead, let's start again from the beginning and see if it's right. That is key. It goes back to me as a 16-year-old – if you don't have the correct diagnosis, then you might be giving incorrect

"THE MORE INFORMATION WE HAVE ABOUT A PERSON'S BODY, THE BETTER."

treatment. I'm also in favour of as many diagnostic tests as possible. The more information we have about a person's body and how it is functioning, the better. My advice to patients is that if a diagnostic test is offered to you, then please take it.

Often the patients I see already have the correct diagnosis and, in that case, I will come up with a different treatment plan. I'm not disagreeing with the way that previous therapists have treated the condition, but I want to try something different.

The way I approach a client with severe chronic pain is that I ask them to tell me what they want to achieve or regain. What's the first thing they need back in their life? Often when they answer, the first part is usually about the pain, but their real desire comes afterwards: 'I just want this pain to go away. I want a good night's sleep,' or, 'I wish I'd never ridden that motorbike. I just want to be able to walk without pain again.'

Once I know what a patient's main priority is, and have the correct diagnosis, I can then start organizing the right doctors or team for them. If you're suffering from severe chronic pain, take a moment to think about what it is that you want back in your life and make sure that when it comes to treatment, you tell every medical professional and therapist what that is.

Unfortunately, when it's not dealt with, chronic pain usually gets worse. The client often has the means of controlling the pain through painkillers or steroid injections, but it still lingers and it's always going to come back, with the anticipation sometimes just as bad as the pain itself. There is a limitation to these methods of management and only so long that they will help. But you don't have to live with chronic pain. By looking at the

IS THERE SUCH A THING AS HEALTHY PAIN?

whole picture, finding the right diagnosis and treatment, and changing your lifestyle in small ways, you can go on to live pain-free.

HEALTHY PAIN

"

'No pain, no gain!'
'Feel the burn!'
'Push through the pain!'

"

We've all heard these phrases shouted at us by a cheery instructor or read them on a fitness app, but are they true? When do we know to push through the pain? Is there such a thing as *healthy* pain?

To be able to discuss this, we need to be clear on what is *discomfort* and what is actual *pain*. Discomfort is the first thing we might feel when we start a new exercise: it's a shock to the system and our bodies try to adapt quickly to what we're asking them to do. It's also what we might feel a day after we have finished a training session. This is a low-level soreness or ache that is the result of micro-tears in the muscles and tendons and is also referred to as Delayed Onset Muscle Soreness (DOMS). This is actually beneficial, as when the muscle repairs it builds back stronger, gradually increasing the strength of the muscle. DOMS usually occurs a day, or even a couple of days, after exercising, so if the ache you are feeling is during or immediately after exercise then it's unlikely to be DOMS.

If the pain you are feeling is a healthy pain, how can you reduce its impact? The best way to do this is to warm up well and take the time to cool down after exercising. Some of the athletes I work with will spend twenty minutes to one hour warming up as they know how important it is to lessen the chance of an injury. This is not something I'd expect of most people, but ten minutes spent warming up and cooling down can have a huge impact on alleviating healthy aches and preventing injuries.

Another way to reduce discomfort is to change your training. This is not a weakness; this is being smart. Consistent training is far more important than extreme training. Many people make the mistake of training hard for one session, making themselves really sore, and then lose the will and function to train the next day. I've treated lots of

"I THOUGHT I COULD JUST 'RUN OFF' THE PAIN. I WAS WRONG."

patients who have personal trainers that look the business, all chiselled torso and not an ounce of fat on them, and give their clients such a hard workout. 'Keep on going. Push through it!' The clients keep on going and injure themselves.

Finally, the most important thing is that after the exercise, we make time to give our bodies the space to recover and receive all the benefits of the session.

When I was 16 years old and tore my first muscle, I thought I could just 'run off' the pain. I was wrong. This is why the T for **T**ype, in STOP, is so important. We need to assess the *type* of pain, as some need our immediate attention.

If I'd had a pain scale and STOP back when I was 16 years old, I would have known that I'd done some serious damage. I would have rated my pain as a five and realized that the type of pain was a 'stabbing' one, that there was 'weakness in the limb' and 'violent cramping sensations'. I would have known not to continue my training a week later, despite others telling me to do so.

Always refer to your pain scale and STOP. If the pain is a three or over, you can't push through it. If it's a three or four, rest it for a few days or rest between workouts. If you decide to try the same exercise again, do it gradually. Instead of doing fifteen reps, do two and massage the area, and then do another two, all the time assessing those pain levels. Or if you hurt yourself playing a racket sport such as tennis or badminton, take a short break and stretch it out. If the pain still comes back, then you should stop playing. Take a few days away from it, making sure to do lots of stretching in between. If you try again, go back slowly. If you are still feeling the same pain, then you are now entering a five as you can't do the activities you normally enjoy. It's time to seek medical help and there is a later chapter on who you should go to depending on your injury.

As you can see, 'push through the pain' is not something you should be listening to. But what other myths and misconceptions are there around pain? I can tell you now that there are many.

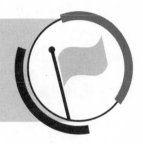

ALWAYS KEEP IN MIND THAT...
there are several types of pain that are warning flags and you should stop exercising immediately if you feel any of the following occur:

- Sharp pain

- Stabbing pain

- A sudden onset of pain

- Persistent pain, where the severity of the pain is getting worse

- Pain at the same site as a previous injury

- Pain on a past surgery site

- Sharp pain when you move part of the body

- A limited range of movement

- You can't move an area of your body

- Weakness in a limb, such as your leg giving way

- Pins and needles that come on suddenly, and are getting worse

- Violent cramping sensations

CHAPTER 2

Myths and Misconceptions

Liam was one of my first patients when I opened my practice doors and I'm lucky to now call him a friend. He'd had a successful business as a tiler for nearly fifteen years, but pain in his back was threatening his ability to work another twenty. His lower back had been aching for a few years and had recently increased to a four and then a five on our pain scale. He kept on taking painkillers to get through his working day, but knew if he wanted to keep tiling until retirement, he was going to have to change something. He had put his discomfort down partly to age and reaching his early forties, as he knew he wasn't a spring chicken any more – tilers younger than him could work a twelve-hour day and not feel a thing the following morning. He used to be one of them.

I was 23 years old when I met Liam, and had just opened the doors to my first clinic. Out in the big wide world, I was looking forward to helping as many people as possible. It was all down to me when it came to treating Liam; there wasn't a helpful tutor to answer my questions any more. During the day, I would spend hours deliberating over which massage table to buy and then I'd read through my university textbooks into the early hours to refresh my knowledge. I'd prepared for months and stocked the shelves with everything I could possibly need – I was finally ready to meet my first patients.

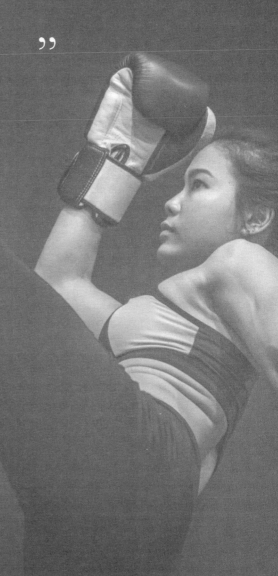

"
Our bodies were designed to move
in a variety of ways.

"

I had anticipated many situations I would face in those early months, but hadn't realized how much of my time would be spent unravelling my clients' incorrect ideas around pain. Those beliefs were deeply instilled, and some had even come from other therapists. It seemed that nearly everyone I treated had at least one misconception about pain, so my practice was based as much on dispelling incorrect ideas as instilling new ones.

It's therefore essential that we start off on the right foot when discussing pain, so I'd like to go through the most common myths

"I'D LIKE TO GO THROUGH THE MOST COMMON MYTHS AND MISCONCEPTIONS SURROUNDING PAIN."

and misconceptions surrounding it and introduce you to a few of the patients I have treated over the years – you might even meet someone with a similar condition to yours.

PATIENT FILES: IS PAIN PART OF GETTING OLD?

When Liam had finished telling me about the pain he was feeling, we ran through the background to his pain in a similar way to STOP. When we got to what **P**rovoked it, I asked Liam to show me how he worked when he was tiling. He crouched down on his knees and motioned the tiling action for me. This was the key point for unlocking his case. After five minutes of watching him, I knew that his pain had nothing to do with ageing. When he was kneeling, he twisted his back, bending and rotating to the side, resulting in one side of his back muscles lengthening while the other shortened.

The reason he was in pain was because he was overworking a muscle called the quadratus lumborum (QL muscle), which is a muscle deep in the back that helps to stabilize your body. I've always believed that people need to understand their bodies so they can understand their pain, so I showed him a diagram of the muscle (see Figure 2.1), allowing him to see for himself how large and integral the QL muscle is to the structure of our backs.

Once I'd helped Liam back up from the floor, we delved into his medical history. When he was in his late twenties, he had been in an accident and injured the middle section of his back, which is responsible for helping us twist. Adults have thirty-three vertebrae along their spines with the sacrum and coccyx bones being fused, and he had fractured his T12 vertebra. (As a side note, you can fracture a bone in your back and not end up paralysed. Paralysis happens when the spinal cord, which the vertebrae protect, is damaged.) Liam had hurt an area of his back that was responsible for twisting, so his body had tried to fix this by asking the lower part of his back to compensate.

Liam had to treat his work as if he was an athlete and his job was his chosen sport. He needed to warm up for it in the morning and take regular breaks to stretch out. He also started strengthening exercises for the QL muscle, including daily squats and mobility exercises, such as thoracic rotations, in the morning before work. Throughout his day, he had been leaning more to his left, so he needed to stretch more towards his right when he did some of his exercises – it's all about rebalancing the body. His back pain gradually lessened, and he was able to continue working as a tiler.

Like Liam, many people believe it is natural to have pain as you grow older. It's true that as you age your body naturally begins to deteriorate as you're more susceptible to injuries, worn cartilage, and joint problems. If you had an MRI scan on your back in your early thirties it would probably show some degeneration. Patients often hear this and decide that it's all downhill for them. However, what they don't know is that if you scanned the back of a Premiership footballer or an Olympic athlete at the same age, they would have degeneration too. However, and this is key, with daily exercises and stretches your body should carry you well into your later years before anything starts to give you pain. Therefore, please don't expect pain as a consequence

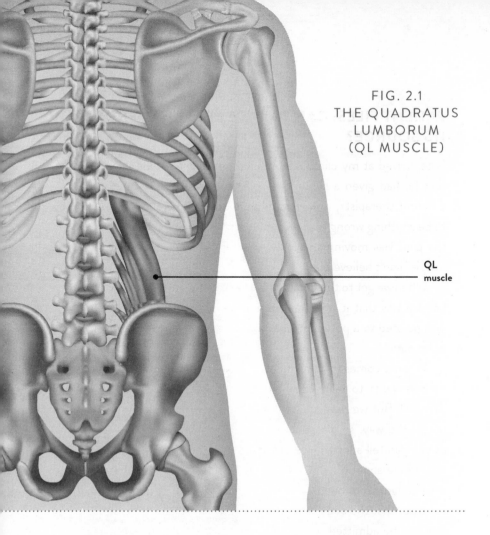

FIG. 2.1
THE QUADRATUS
LUMBORUM
(QL MUSCLE)

QL
muscle

of getting older. It's a message from your body that something isn't quite right. It all goes back to our bodies being designed to *move* in a *variety* of ways and if we don't fulfil these basic requirements then pain eventually lets us know that something isn't working properly.

In Liam's case, he had an active job but his back pain stemmed from repeating the same action over and over again. Our bodies are not designed for repetition of the same movement for eight hours a day, five days a week. They were designed for walking several hours a day, while bending occasionally to dig up a tasty root vegetable or stretching for some berries. Like Liam, most of us can't easily change our professions. If this isn't a possibility, we should try to make time for stretches and exercises that balance out the demands placed on our bodies. There is more on this in the later chapters.

PATIENT FILES: CAN PAIN BE FELT AWAY FROM ITS SOURCE?

Pete arrived at my clinic with constant pain in his right shoulder that he had given a six on the pain scale. He had been to see different therapists, who were all perplexed as there didn't seem to be anything wrong with his shoulder; the tissue felt healthy and the joint was moving smoothly. He was beginning to wonder if people didn't believe him.

When we got to the Onset of his pain, he told me that the daily pattern was that it worsened in the evening after he had eaten. This pointed to a potential digestion issue, but was this the cause of his pain?

When it comes to digestion, there is a key bit of evidence that no one wants to talk about because it's too embarrassing, too personal. But we have to say it: stools! There we go, we've got it out of the way, so please don't gloss over this if someone asks, as you can tell a lot from them about how the body is working. I asked Pete about his, and he told me they floated. This can mean several things, but one is that they might contain a lot of fat, which indicates that the body isn't absorbing nutrients. I asked about his diet and he admitted to regularly eating junk food. When he lay down on the table, I went straight to the site where I thought the problem might be and palpated the area around his gallbladder. He felt an immediate burst of pain that he rated as an eight and I was certain I knew what the problem was – he had gallstones. The next day he went to see his doctor, who confirmed the diagnosis. They were soon removed, leaving Pete with no more pain in his shoulder.

'Referred pain' is a term you will hopefully become familiar with. It's when pain is felt in an area of the body that is not where the injury or disease is, and it's very common (see Figure 2.2). The opposite to this is 'primary pain', when you feel pain at the source of the injury or condition. In Pete's case, his gallbladder was enlarged from the

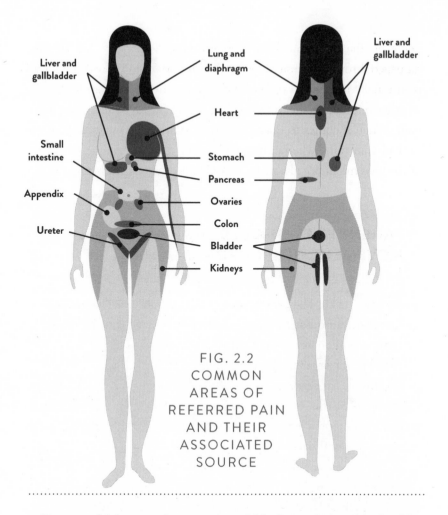

Liver and
gallblader

Lung and
diaphragm

Liver and
gallbladder

Small
intestine

Heart

Appendix

Stomach

Ureter

Pancreas

Ovaries

Colon

Bladder

Kidneys

FIG. 2.2
COMMON
AREAS OF
REFERRED PAIN
AND THEIR
ASSOCIATED
SOURCE

gallstones, which pressed on a nerve, which shot pain into his shoulder. Put simply, the pain was masquerading as tissue damage to his shoulder (or put less simply, it was somatic nociceptive pain, if you want the medical terminology from Figure 1.1 in Chapter 1). However, his pain was actually caused by damage to one of his organs, which led to nerve pain (visceral nociceptive pain leading to peripheral neuropathic pain – it's all there in Figure 1.1!) This is quite common, and people can also feel pain in their shoulder from damage to their liver or heart as well.

Another common type of referred pain, and one you have probably heard of, is sciatica. This is a generalized term for lower-back pain, but the pain often shoots down the leg as well. It's caused by a disc pressing on a nerve in the lower back. Either the pain can come from a trapped nerve on the route out of the spinal cord, or a nerve has become damaged through trauma or disease. It's important to know that referred pain usually indicates a damaged or trapped nerve, so always consider whether your pain is shooting, tingling, or burning, as these suggest nerve pain. When it comes to diagnosing your own pain, always have in the back of your mind whether it could be referred pain – that is, the source of the pain might not always be as straightforward as you first thought.

PATIENT FILES: SHOULD I RESTRICT MY MOVEMENT WITH CHRONIC PAIN?

Sonia had come to me with back pain, as probably two thirds of my patients do. The back is a complex structure as it has multiple functions. It houses the spinal cord, which is the main channel of communication between the brain and other areas of the body. It contains our organs, and holds them in the right place. It is also responsible for carrying our weight and allows us to move flexibly. On top of all this, our backs are expected to compensate when we lose movement in other areas. As with all things, the more complex something is, the more things there are that can go wrong.

Sonia was in her forties and spent her days standing as she worked in a shop. She had a constant dull ache in the lower part of her back and had difficulty sleeping because of it. When we got to the Onset of the pain, she mentioned that it had started a few months after she had begun lying down on her sofa every evening to watch TV. I asked her why she had started doing this, as it was likely that something had changed if she had formed a new habit. That's when she told me she lay down because she was scared to *sit* down. This clearly needed more questioning. Eventually it came out that a few years earlier she'd had a fall and damaged the cartilage in her knee. She'd had minor keyhole surgery, whereby the knee was washed out, but there was no aftercare and she couldn't bend her knee because of a sharp pain. It was now perfectly understandable that she was afraid to sit down.

I treat the body as a whole, so I looked at her knee straightaway because the back pain was effectively a symptom of the knee. She'd adjusted her lifestyle and it had caused a separate issue. After inspecting her knee, I knew it was treatable. If I loosened her quadriceps, which are the large muscles in the thigh that I had torn when I was 16 years old, and the popliteus at the back of the knee, she would get her knee function back. She could then bend her knee to sit down and her back could begin to recover from all those years of damage that lying on her couch had done.

> "I TREAT THE BODY AS A WHOLE, SO I LOOKED AT HER KNEE STRAIGHT AWAY BECAUSE THE BACK PAIN WAS EFFECTIVELY A SYMPTOM OF THE KNEE."

Sonia's case is a common one as there is often limited aftercare following surgery or an injury. It's completely understandable that she curled up on her couch in the evenings, because what do we do when we're in pain? We restrict out movement, curl up, and try to protect ourselves. It's instinctive. If Sonia had been given the right exercises following her surgery, it's very likely she wouldn't have had pain in her knee. She then wouldn't have tried to adapt to this by lying down in the evenings and her back wouldn't have been injured.

Nowadays, it's very rare that people are told by medical professionals not to try physiotherapy after surgery or an injury, but if that is the case, then always go by what your doctor is telling you. Normally, you will be given exercises to do, but this isn't always as useful as having someone to do them with. If you can't afford a therapist, then ask a family member or friend to do the exercises with you on a regular basis.

Even if you can't exercise the area, it doesn't always mean that you must stop all types of exercise. It's good to load your other joints as it releases hormones that help your mood and reminds your brain that you are still able to move. If the pain is in your lower half, then lift some light weights with your top half, and vice versa. If the pain is in your back, try having a gentle go on an exercise bike and see how that feels. Keep your body moving if you can, because that is what it is designed to do.

PATIENT FILES: SHOULD I JUST LIVE WITH PAIN?

Jamie loved Thai kickboxing, so much so that he had a coach. When I first met him, he was in his thirties and had pulled his adductor muscle, which is in the inner thigh. This meant he didn't have a full range of movement in his hip. He hadn't trained for a month and was scared he was going to hurt himself again.

For years he'd been feeling pain in his hip. He'd mentioned it several times to his coach, who had told him that it was normal to feel pain in kickboxing and he had to keep going. Being a dutiful student, and questioning whether his own pain thresholds were lower than everyone around him, he kept on going. One day in training he did a high kick and then collapsed on the floor. Pain was tired of politely knocking at his door.

If Jamie had a pain scale and STOP, he would have realized that even though his pain was a two it was in fact chronic pain, because it always returned to the same site and was the same type of pain. He would then have seen a therapist who would have realized that the source of his pain was a muscle in his hip flexor called the psoas muscle, which was tight. They would have released the tension there and the injury to his adductor muscle would have been prevented.

If there is only one message you take from this book, it is that you should never battle through your pain.

PATIENT FILES: IS MEDICATION FOR LIFE?

People who try and battle through pain often rely on painkillers and Charlotte had been taking them for nearly two years when she first came through my door. She had recently started taking diazepam as well, which is prescription-only and can be highly addictive. It's not classed as a painkiller, but is used to treat muscle spasms. Most people know it by one of its brand names – Valium.

Charlotte was suffering from pain in her shoulder and wrist, and had also lost the grip in her hand. She had been advised to take painkillers, but the root of the problem hadn't yet been found. She was now worried about using diazepam for a long period of time, but had been prescribed it for the problem with her arms. The alternative wasn't particularly appealing either. Years of taking paracetamol and ibuprofen had made them ineffective, as she had built up a resistance to them.

When we got to the Type of pain, she told me it could be shooting, which is a clear sign of nerve pain. I asked her to take me through her average day and quickly realized that she spent a lot of time on a motorbike. When we imagine a biker or a serious cyclist, we probably envisage them hunched over handlebars, their shoulders rolled in. Our bodies are not meant to be held like this for long periods, and it was therefore likely that this was the root cause of her pain.

After I had examined her, I realized she had a condition called thoracic outlet syndrome in which the bundle of nerves in the shoulder, called the brachial plexus, are compressed. Her posture on the motorbike had caused this. These nerve branches from the spinal cord help control movement and sensation in the arm and hand. This vital bundle of nerves can often get trapped in the collarbone, scalene muscle, or even in the first rib, which is just above your collarbone (see Figure 2.3).

I did some work to loosen the pressure from the collarbone and the front of her neck. The aim was to open out her chest, which

I have to do with many of my clients, as we hunch and curl in on ourselves, particularly when we are in pain, which exacerbates so many conditions. Charlotte's shoulders were rolled in from riding the motorbike and she needed to open up. She carried on with the stretches at home and initially limited the amount of time she spent on her bike. Eventually, if she stretched before using her bike, she was able to ride it as often as she used to.

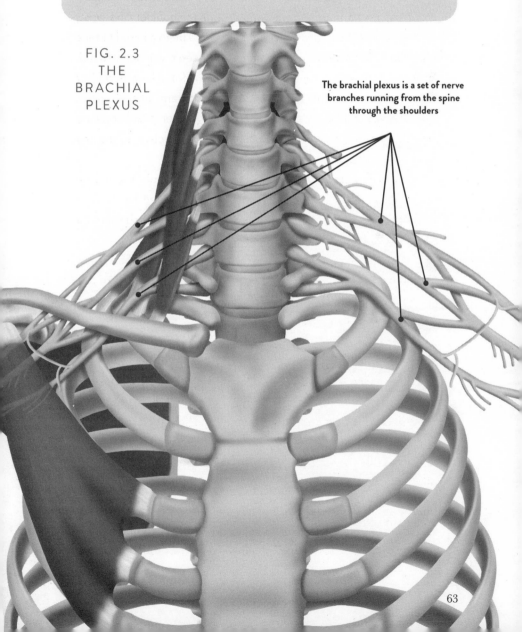

FIG. 2.3
THE
BRACHIAL
PLEXUS

The brachial plexus is a set of nerve branches running from the spine through the shoulders

For many people, painkillers are a daily ritual and for some, their usage can quickly get out of control. I have seen several patients who have started off using opioid painkillers as a way of numbing their pain, only to become addicted. Even if clients rely on less addictive painkillers, such as paracetamol or ibuprofen, the medication's ability to numb begins to reduce the more you take them. Painkillers also have many side effects, which I discuss in Chapter 16. They might be useful in providing short-term relief, but in most of the cases I see they should be approached with caution for long-term use. Rehabilitation can often ease the need for painkillers and should usually be the starting point when considering treatment.

PATIENT FILES: IT'S ALL IN YOUR HEAD

Sarah was another of my early patients and I first met her when she was in her fifties. She had sat hunched in on herself as she quietly told me she had pain in her shoulder. When it came to her past medical history, she informed me that she'd been diagnosed with chronic fatigue and fibromyalgia. She then quickly looked up to watch my reaction to this news. Unfortunately, they are both conditions for which patients used to be told that the pain they were feeling was psychological. Both conditions can cause all-over body pain and Sarah confirmed that she suffered from aches throughout her body and always felt tired. For years she had been told that there was no physical reason for the pain in her shoulder; and she had also been taking anti-depressants for over five years.

Chronic fatigue (also known as ME – which stands for myalgic encephalomyelitis) and fibromyalgia are both very misunderstood and it has only been in the last few years that chronic fatigue has no longer been classified as a psychological disease. I knew that when it came to treating Sarah, I needed to take a 360-degree, holistic approach. I began by tackling the pain in her shoulder and set about loosening the tense muscles there.

As I worked, I noticed that her posture was poor and that her shoulders were pulled in towards her chest. She'd had several setbacks in previous years, and it was almost as if the emotional pain of what she had experienced had started to have physical consequences. She pulled herself in, sheltering herself from the world. I knew then that she might benefit from some lifestyle changes and hopefully begin to unfurl.

Previous practitioners had only treated her shoulder, but because of stress and anxiety her ribs and abdomen were tight. I gave her some exercises so she could practise opening up her chest. She began to feel their benefit and in later appointments we began to discuss her sleep and how massage could help. Soon she had more energy and was suffering less from this mixture of all three types of pain. I loosened up her shoulder and because she wasn't hunching in on herself any more, the pain there didn't come back again. Her sleep improved and consequently her mood lifted. Also, because she had improved her posture and opened up her chest, the general aches she was feeling also lessened and didn't return to their previous levels.

Pain is complex as it involves both the body and the mind. The psychological suffering that comes with physical pain can certainly make us more miserable, and dwelling on the pain can make us lose hope of it getting better. It can also make us afraid of movement or performing daily tasks. Also, some types of psychological suffering can bring about real feelings of physical pain. It's therefore important for therapists and doctors to have empathy when they gather all the information from the patient.

It's also important to remember that scans, such as an MRI, don't always show the entire picture. Even some of the professional athletes I've worked with have been told that their pain is not real as scans show no abnormality. Please don't think that if an MRI or other scan comes back showing that everything is fine, that is the end of the matter and the pain therefore shouldn't exist. I've heard about so many patients who count down the days until a scan, hoping that they will finally have some answers, and then it comes back clear. What they don't know is that a scan can't pick up an imbalance or the tonal quality of the muscle, which can instead be checked by running your hands over it. Scans are a good reference point and can show when further investigations are needed, but they are not always the final answer.

PATIENT FILES: IT'S BETTER NOT TO FEEL PAIN

Lyall was in his early sixties when he came to me with lower-back pain. Whenever clients have lower-back pain, I instantly start to consider whether it's affecting other areas, as there are so many nerves that travel through this area. I therefore began by examining Lyall's legs and when I came to his feet, I noticed he had a foot drop (see Figure 2.4). He was sitting on my therapy table with his legs dangling over the end and couldn't move his foot upwards by ninety degrees so his toes pointed straight ahead.

I mentioned this to him, and he confirmed that he was constantly tripping over things as his foot couldn't clear the floor. This is the classic outcome of a foot drop and something that can be very dangerous for obvious reasons. The loss of power and sensation in the foot meant he was dragging his right foot on the ground, and

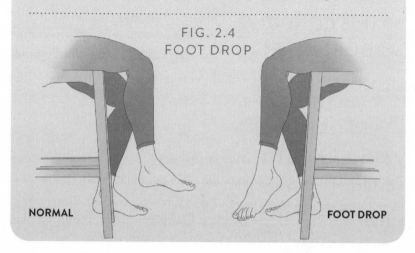

FIG. 2.4
FOOT DROP

NORMAL   FOOT DROP

he was off balance because his foot was numb. He then showed me how he could pinch the skin on his foot and not feel a thing. He had wished his back was like that as well.

It may not come as a surprise that I didn't feel exactly the same as Lyall about his back, but I could understand his point of view. The pain he had been feeling in his back was stopping him from sleeping and he was feeling desperate because of it. I examined his lower back and suspected he had multiple disc bulges, which were later confirmed by an MRI scan. The foot drop was actually a symptom of the disc bulge pressing on a nerve in his lower back. I treated him by taking the pressure off the nerve, but the bulk of his recovery was down to him. He needed to do daily exercises to get the muscle firing and teach the brain that he could use it again. He kept up with the exercises and soon his foot drop was resolved.

Lyall's case of being unable to feel pain was localized to his foot, but there are extreme cases of people who have never felt pain in any part of their bodies. These are congenital cases, meaning the condition exists from birth. Fortunately, they are very rare and are usually the result of a genetic issue. People with this condition can put their hands in a pan of boiling water and don't feel a thing; they can jump down a flight of stairs and either land safely or not feel their fibula snap. Some people might view this as almost having a superpower, but it actually severely reduces life expectancy. There is the obvious outcome that people with this condition are unable to react to the messages that their bodies are telling them to try and help the healing process. But there is another more serious consequence. As

"IN PARTICULAR, YOUNG MEN WITH THIS CONDITION ARE OFTEN PRONE TO EXTREME STUNTS THAT UNFORTUNATELY EITHER KILL THEM, OR THEY SUFFER LIFE-CHANGING INJURIES."

children, pain teaches us caution and we slowly learn the boundaries of what we can do without hurting ourselves. If someone doesn't have this restriction tugging them back when they are young, then they can often take huge risks, even into their adult years. In particular, young men with this condition are prone to extreme stunts that unfortunately either kill them, or result in life-changing injuries.

A much more common case of being unable to feel pain, and one I have seen several times in my practice is when people in the later stages of diabetes lose the sensation in their feet. This can lead to infections, bruises, blisters, and sprains.

Another thing to be aware of when not feeling pain is the temporary loss of touch or sensation. Because it is temporary, it is known as an 'impaired sensation' and can produce numbness, tingling, or weakness in the area and is very common in people with a disc pressing on a nerve in their lower back. It might not be a classic feeling of 'pain', but once you start making adaptations because of it, then it's a clear sign that it needs to be investigated by a medical professional.

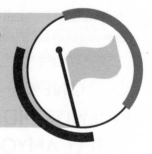

IMPAIRED SENSATION CAN ...

sometimes signal a serious neurological condition, such as a stroke, so always seek immediate medical attention if you suddenly experience any of the following:

- **Loss of balance or dizziness**
- **Confusion**
- **Severe headache**
- **Weakness in the body**
- **Changes to your vision**

The prostate is a small walnut-sized gland that is located between the penis and bladder. It helps make semen and is part of men's reproductive system. Over the years, I have seen several men in my clinic with clear signs of prostate cancer, whom I have referred to their doctor, who later diagnosed it. This is a really important issue to me as many men don't seem to know the warning signs, and if caught early it can often be managed well with a low chance of recurrence. One of my friends didn't tell anyone that he had been peeing blood for three years, and by the time he was diagnosed with prostate cancer, it was too late. Therefore, please keep a watchful eye out for the common signs below:

> "ONE OF MY FRIENDS DIDN'T TELL ANYONE AND BY THE TIME HE WAS DIAGNOSED WITH PROSTATE CANCER IT WAS TOO LATE."

COMMON SIGNS OF PROSTATE CANCER

- **FREQUENT**
  need to urinate, particularly
  during the night

- **PERSISTENT**
  lower back pain, especially if
  over the age of 55

- **DIFFICULTY**
  starting to urinate, or stopping

- **ERECTILE**
  dysfunction

- **BLOOD**
  in urine or semen

- **PAINFUL**
  burning sensation when urinating

SURGERY IS THE BEST OPTION

Someone I wish I'd been able to treat was myself when I was 16 years old. At that time, I had decided to have surgery after tearing a muscle in my thigh, but I now know that rehabilitation can often lessen pain without surgery.

I want to make it clear that I am not against surgery. Surgery is a lifesaver, a restorer of movement, and often a reliever of pain. The advances in surgery over the past 200 years are among the key things that have moved medicine into the modern era. However, surgery is often viewed as a 'quick fix' and if someone is facing it, they should try to consider all the possible outcomes and side effects. It's important that, if you decide to go down the surgical route, the specialist explains in detail the aftercare of the surgery. In my experience many patients don't know what to do after surgery in terms of exercising and rehabilitation, and these are often key to the surgery's success.

So, if I had a young man come through my door, trying to brush off the pain and telling me he would be back running again the following week, I'd firstly have run through STOP. My **T**ype of pain was a deep ache, and this would have been more likely to come from tissue instead of nerve damage. I would then introduce him to RICE, which is a commonly used mnemonic for treating tissue damage and is the first treatment we will learn about:

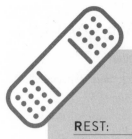

R - I - C - E
To treat tissue damage

REST:

Don't try and 'run off' the injury. Instead, rest it until you've done further investigations and know what you are dealing with.

ICE:

Anything ice-cold wrapped in a tea towel will do – frozen peas are always a popular option.

COMPRESSION:

This is wrapping a bandage around the area to help reduce swelling, which in turn will help reduce the pain. You can now buy self-adhesive bandages so there's no need for pins, or the right size of elasticated tube bands.

ELEVATION:

This means lifting a limb slightly higher than the heart. It helps blood flow, drains excess fluid, reduces swelling, and therefore helps reduce pain.

The above is your general starting point for treating tissue damage and one that you should try to remember. Next, I would have touched the area lightly and felt a possible tear in the quad muscle. In my experience, light massage to a torn muscle can help begin the process of muscle realignment, but should only be done by someone trained in it, as it can make the tear deeper if done incorrectly. I find that dry needling also really helps with muscle tears. Most importantly, a muscle tear should be given time to heal as not doing so is what usually leads to the tear getting worse, or in very rare cases, results in calcified tissue.

I always look at the body as a whole and would therefore have realized that the pain in my lower back was the original source of the injury. It was tight and putting pressure on the hip joint, meaning that the quad muscle needed to work harder, which led to it tearing. All three of these areas needed to be treated.

Even if my 16-year-old self had faced either surgery or steroid injections, owing to calcified tissue, I would have chosen the injections. In my experience, electroacupuncture can break down calcified tissue or bring function back into the muscle. As I've said before, steroid injections aren't a permanent fix, but they would have provided me with more time for treatment, reduced the inflammation, and hopefully returned full movement to the muscle. I now know that it doesn't matter if the calcified tissue is there, as long as the muscle functions. I think I could have lived with that.

Now that we all have a basic understanding of pain and the common misconceptions surrounding it, it's time to move on to Part Two of this book, which is all about diagnosis and treatment.

PART TWO

Parts of the Body: Diagnosis and Treatment

CHAPTER 3

From Head
to Toe

In this section I cover the most common types of injuries, ailments, and diseases I see in my practice and how they are diagnosed – starting at the head and working our way down to the toes. If you have a good grounding in what might be wrong, you can then select the right medical professional or therapist to see, know the right questions to ask, and begin to think about what treatment you might need. If it is a less serious injury, then you might even begin to treat yourself at home. As with all things, trust your instincts. If you believe that something requires urgent medical attention or if you are worried about something, then you should contact your doctor or another medical professional.

But, before we get into the specifics for each area of the body, there are a few things that you should be aware of when it comes to diagnosing the most common conditions. These apply to all areas of the body and are designed to help you with your diagnosis and not to replace a diagnosis from a medical professional.

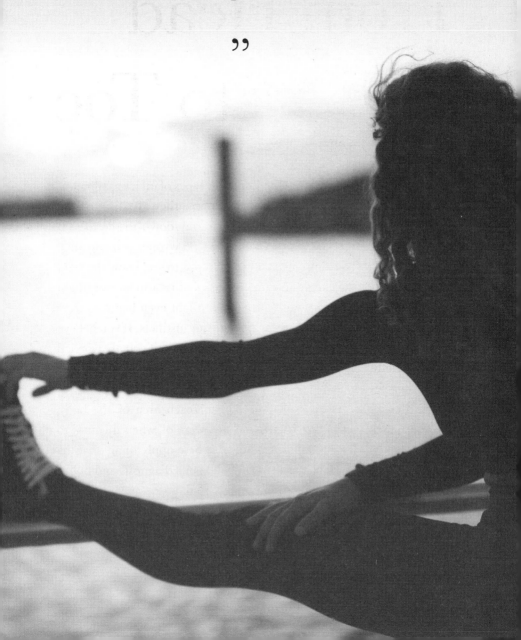

> "
> If you are worried about
> something, then you should contact
> a medical professional.
> "

MUSCLE STRAINS AND MUSCLE TEARS

You have felt a sharp pain when exercising, or perhaps a gradual ache has been increasing over the last few days. You have run through your pain scale and STOP and believe that it is tissue damage because of the **T**ype of pain and the **O**nset, but you're unsure whether it's a potential strain or a tear. The two can easily be confused. This is what happened to one of my clients, Tim, who thought he'd strained his hamstring muscle while playing squash. The pain was only around a five on the pain scale, and because of this he didn't think it could be a tear. He therefore carried on trying to play squash with a small tear over the next week before seeing me.

There is a grey area around muscle strains and tears as an extreme strain can overlap with a tear, but generally speaking we can differentiate between the two. A muscle *strain*, or *pulled muscle* as it is sometimes called, is when a muscle has been overworked but there is no long-lasting damage, whereas a muscle *tear* is clearly a much more serious condition. Muscle strains usually happen in the legs or back and occur when the fibres that make up our muscles are overstretched, or worked too hard or too fast.

Muscle tears are more serious because the tissue has separated and needs rest or possibly surgery to repair it. Like burns, muscle tears are graded. The grading of the tear is usually determined by an MRI scan. The grading is important because if you have suffered a complete tear then you will most likely need surgery, whereas you should recover from a mild tear in a couple of weeks. If it's a partial tear you might also be offered surgery, but that isn't always the only option. I've helped 40–60 per cent tears recover completely with the right treatment and rehabilitation, without the need for surgery.

The first thing to do when diagnosing a recent potential tear is to check if the area is swollen, warm, red, or puffy. All of these are indications of inflammation, which is the body's rapid response to tissue damage such as a tear. Usually, with a strain there won't be any inflammation, so the area will look and feel the same when you touch it. If there is warmth and swelling, then use **R**est, **I**ce, **C**ompression, and **E**levation to treat it.

GRADINGS OF TEARS
TEARS ARE USUALLY GRADED 1–3

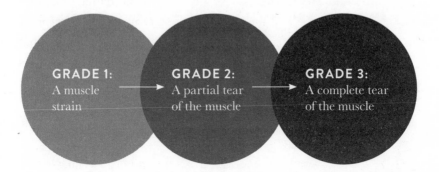

GRADE 1: A muscle strain → **GRADE 2:** A partial tear of the muscle → **GRADE 3:** A complete tear of the muscle

A few years ago, when I was working there, British Athletics developed a new, more detailed grading system that is now widely used in the sporting world. It scores a muscle injury between zero and four. It's more comprehensive than the one to three scale as, in my opinion, Grade two from the old system is too broad. A detailed explanation of how the depth and position of the tear affects the grading is beyond the remit of this book, but in brief, the grading is as follows:

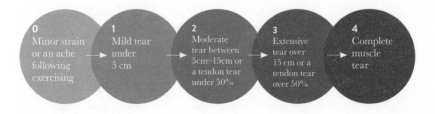

0 Minor strain or an ache following exercising → **1** Mild tear under 5 cm → **2** Moderate tear between 5cm–15cm or a tendon tear under 50% → **3** Extensive tear over 15 cm or a tendon tear over 50% → **4** Complete muscle tear

One of the most simplistic ways of deciding if a muscle is torn or strained is that usually, with a strained muscle, you can still use it and the pain doesn't alter. With a muscle tear, the pain normally increases when it is moved. This isn't a guarantee, as there are always anomalies, but generally speaking, if the pain doesn't increase if you move the muscle then it's more likely to be a strain. A strain will still be painful and there may even be mild weakness in the area, but with a tear there will be swelling and redness if it happened in the past few days.

? **WHAT IS A MUSCLE SPASM?**
Muscle spasms can affect anyone, regardless of age or fitness level. They happen in all areas of the body and occur when the muscle contracts involuntarily. Stretching and massage can help, as well as contrast bathing (switching between heat and ice on the area).

Another way of differentiating a tear from a strain is that with a tear you lose power in the muscle and can't contract a muscle fully, so will naturally try and leave it in a resting position.

From experience, I can often feel a strain or tear to a muscle, but would only use that as part of a diagnosis and would gather other information such as testing the muscle, the case history, STOP, the pain level and, if necessary, an MRI scan. You shouldn't just use one response to decide on a diagnosis, as it's better to have as much information as you can before making that decision. Therefore, try and gather as much evidence as you can before considering whether it is a strain or a tear.

TENDONS AND LIGAMENTS

My client, Marcus, ran three times a week and had started getting pain in his knee. He'd been to a therapist who told him it was likely to be his IT band, which is a thick band of tissue that runs up the outside of your thigh and helps stabilize the knee. He'd been told to massage it at home with a foam roller. A month later the pain was getting worse and there was swelling. By the time he came to me it was clear that he had damaged a ligament in his knee. But what is the job of a ligament and how does it differ from a tendon?

As you can see in Figure 3.1, tendons are connective tissues located at the end of a muscle and attach the muscle to a bone. Ligaments are also made from fibrous tissue, but they attach bone to bone, helping stabilize the bones and making sure they don't go beyond the range of a joint.

You can tear or strain either a ligament or a tendon. If a ligament is strained it is called a 'sprain', so if someone has sprained their ankle, they have pulled a ligament in their ankle, not a muscle. If you tear a tendon or ligament, you will often be offered surgery. The **O**nset of the pain will usually be sudden or straight after trauma. Generally, a muscle tear will recover quicker than either a ligament or tendon, because it has such a good blood supply.

Ligaments have their own tearing system, which is graded 1–3: one is a mild partial tear; two is moderate, or midway; and three is a complete tear, which is also known as a 'rupture'. With different physical tests, a therapist or doctor should be able to tell the difference between a ligament and tendon tear. For example, with the cruciate ligament in the knee – or the ligaments around the side of the knee – if they are torn, the knee joint will feel loose, because the ligaments around the joint help stabilize it and are not working as well. Often patients will say their knee has 'given way', or they can't put all their weight on it and it feels floppy. If the patient mentions a *click* or a *pop*, this can often be a sign of a ligament tear. With suspected ligament damage, I gently press the site of where the ligament

FIG. 3.1
TENDONS AND LIGAMENTS

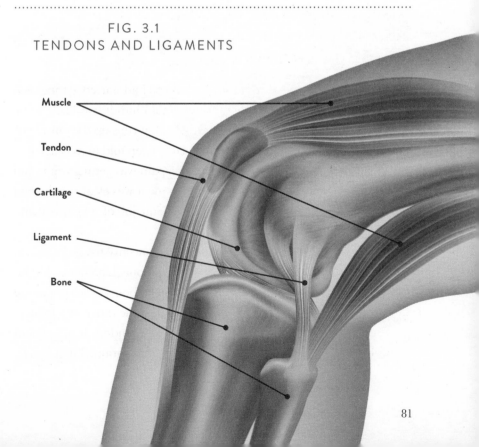

Muscle

Tendon

Cartilage

Ligament

Bone

is located, as an increase in pain will suggest a tear. Damage to a ligament is usually quite straightforward to treat and manage.

A tear to a tendon is similar to a muscle tear in that when the tendon is contracted it will hurt, or will be difficult to contract at all. Damage to a tendon is generally more complicated than a ligament as the tendon is attached to the end of a muscle, whereas a ligament is off by itself holding two bones in place. A tear to a tendon will often cause a dysfunction to the muscle it is attached to as well, because they are so interwoven. Because of this, there are individual ways of treating different tendons as they are each unique depending on which muscle they are attached to.

> **"IF THE PATIENT MENTIONS A *CLICK* OR A *POP*, THIS CAN OFTEN BE A SIGN OF A LIGAMENT TEAR."**

INFLAMMATION

When there is '–itis' at the end of a word it means that there is inflammation. Common examples are tendon*itis* (inflammation of a tendon), bronch*itis* (inflammation of the bronchi in the lungs), and arthritis (inflammation of the joints). Inflammation usually makes an area warm and appear swollen and red. Inflammation is the body's natural immune response to an injury or infection when it is trying to heal the area. Inflammation can cause pain as it swells the area, which is why ice should be applied to try and help reduce the swelling.

BURSAE

We've all heard of muscles, ligaments, tendons, and joints, but quite a few of us probably haven't heard of a 'bursa', which is an area of the body that can suffer from inflammation. These are a fluid-filled pads that are located all over your body and cushion the tissues from too much friction. You have bursae near your large joints such as the knee, elbow, and hips, and even two in your bum to prevent the tissue rubbing against your pelvic bone.

Bursitis is a common condition that many people don't know they have. It happens when a bursa becomes inflamed. The area will normally ache and is more painful when you press on it, which usually happens when there is too much pressure on the bursa, such as from sitting a lot during the day. It will usually be tender, warm, or swollen. It's a localized condition as well, so it is unlikely that you'd have it at the site of multiple joints simultaneously, as you would with rheumatoid arthritis. So, if you experience these symptoms near a joint it might be bursitis and you should contact your doctor as they might need to examine you. Bursitis is difficult to diagnose and can be confused with other conditions, so a scan might be needed for a firm diagnosis.

ARTHRITIS

More than ten million people in the UK have arthritis. It affects the joints in the body and there is no cure but, with the right treatment, it can be managed successfully. The two most common types of arthritis are osteoarthritis and rheumatoid arthritis.

....

- **OSTEOARTHRITIS:**

  Osteoarthritis is the most common type of arthritis and it's estimated that 8.75 million people in the UK suffer from it. Osteoarthritis happens when the cartilage in a joint begins to change, and this leads to the surrounding bone to begin to break down. There is usually joint pain and stiffness. There is no cure, but with the right treatment its progress can be halted. Osteoarthritis is diagnosed through an X-ray.

- **RHEUMATOID ARTHRITIS:**

  Rheumatoid arthritis happens when the immune system starts to attack the healthy cells in the joints. It commonly makes the joint red and swollen and often affects multiple joints at once. You can also suffer from fever and night sweats. There are certain medications such as steroids that can help. The diagnosis for rheumatoid arthritis is through blood tests.

....

I talk about arthritis in several sections of the book as it can affect nearly all the joints. When thinking about arthritis it's always good to consider whether it is rheumatoid arthritis or osteoarthritis, as they usually require different treatment. With both conditions, you should see your doctor for a diagnosis, but can receive treatment from an osteopath or physiotherapist. With rheumatoid arthritis there are other symptoms that should also be considered (see Figure 3.2).

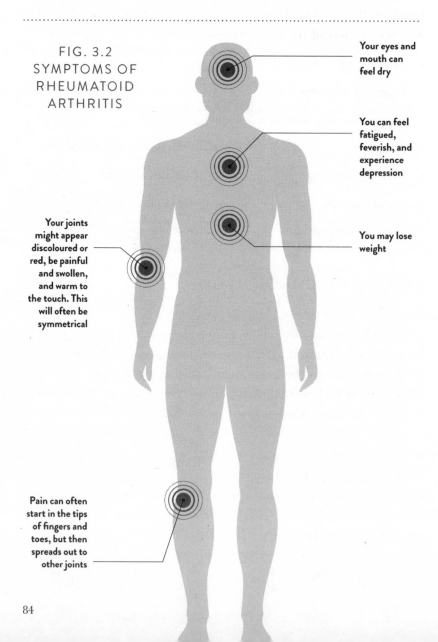

FIG. 3.2
SYMPTOMS OF
RHEUMATOID
ARTHRITIS

Your eyes and mouth can feel dry

You can feel fatigued, feverish, and experience depression

Your joints might appear discoloured or red, be painful and swollen, and warm to the touch. This will often be symmetrical

You may lose weight

Pain can often start in the tips of fingers and toes, but then spreads out to other joints

FEVER

A fever is a raised temperature of 38°C or above. Fevers are a natural part of the immune system's response when fighting infection. They normally last between one and three days and do not usually require treatment. However, if the fever lasts longer than three days and is higher than 39.4°C then this can be a sign of a more serious condition and does require medical attention. Other signs of a more serious condition that need medical attention are if you have a fever together with one or more of the following symptoms:

- dehydration
- breathing difficulties
- confusion or disorientation
- dizziness
- frequent vomiting
- muscle cramps
- urinating infrequently

- pain when urinating
- rash
- seizures
- sensitivity to bright light
- a severe headache
- stiff neck or neck pain
- dark or strong-smelling urine.

ACUTE AND CHRONIC PAIN

Remember when treating an injury to consider whether the pain is acute or chronic as it affects how it should be treated. This is important because if it is *chronic*, it will have lasted more than three months and it's unlikely there will be inflammation. If the injury is *acute*, meaning it's been there for less than three months, and you are trying to treat it in the first few days, it is possible there will also be inflammation.

Injuries with inflammation need to be treated differently from those without. If there is inflammation, don't apply heat as it can slow down the healing process. Instead, apply ice. If the condition is chronic and there are no signs of inflammation (i.e. redness, swelling, or feeling warm to touch), then you can use contrast bathing to treat the area, which is switching between applying heat and ice.

CHAPTER 4

Head

and face

We have over forty muscles in our face which, with just a fleeting look, can help us express our needs, joys, and fears. We use them to chew our food, move our lips to form words and operate the sensory organs that are housed there.

But we also carry a great deal of stress and tension in our face and rarely take the time to treat it. We wash it, maybe put makeup on, but when do we take the time to massage it? Just a simple massage of our face and scalp can help prevent some of the below conditions and is something that can provide relief from pain and discomfort.

SYMPTOMS
CHECK

IS YOUR JAW HEALTHY?

Your healthy jaw should be able to do the following without any pain, clicking, or locking:

1	2	3	4
Open and close your mouth	Move your lower jaw from side to side	Extend your lower jaw forwards so that the bottom teeth are in front of the upper jaw	When you open your mouth, you should be able to fit three sideways fingers between your top and bottom teeth

"

We carry a great deal of
stress and tension in our face.

"

With all these muscles comes a requirement for nerves to spark them into life. There are both *sensory* and *motor* elements to nerves, which function in a similar way to an electricity supply, but in the body – without them, there isn't any movement. If you want to smile a thankyou, you can't do this without the involvement of nerves. Often, with conditions that affect the head and face, there is a mixture of both nerve and tissue pain and both elements need to be considered when treating this area.

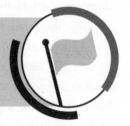

We should be aware of several warning flags when it comes to the head and face, so always seek urgent medical attention if you experience any of the following:

- Headache with a fever or stiff neck
- Unexplained weight loss
- Unexplained nausea or vomiting
- Onset of sudden pain that is like a thunderclap sensation
- Change in a pattern of headaches
- Headaches that happen more regularly and increase in intensity
- A positional headache, which is a headache that changes substantially in intensity when you move
- No previous history of headaches and a new headache that limits some of your normal activities
- Permanent headache
- Stabbing headache
- Headache following trauma
- Slurred speech
- Sudden dizziness or lack of balance
- Numbness or weakness on one side of the face or body
- Sight issues in one or both eyes

MOST COMMON HEAD AND FACE CONDITIONS: HEADACHES

No one can really agree on how many types of headaches there are. Some researchers believe there are twenty-eight, others over a hundred. Fundamentally, it doesn't really matter to the person who is suffering from one of them – they just want to know how they can relieve it. Globally, it is thought that half of all adults have had at least one headache in the past year. The first step is to pinpoint where the pain is being felt, as this can help diagnose which of the eight main types of headaches it is (see Figure 4.1).

Once the type of headache has been identified, it might have an obvious root cause that can be treated, such as a dental, temporomandibular joint (TMJ), neck, or sinus headache, or even simply headaches resulting from dehydration which are very easily fixed. I see a lot of clients with headaches at the top and side of their heads that are the result of the muscles in their neck being tight. Once these are loosened and restored to how they should be, the pain goes away.

FIG. 4.1
MAIN TYPES OF HEADACHE

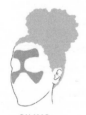 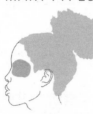 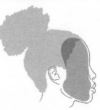 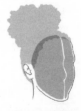

SINUS	**CLUSTER**	**MIGRAINE**	**HORMONAL**
Pressure around the eye, forehead and cheeks.	Felt on only one side of the head, usually around the eye.	Usually only on one side of the head. Often accompanied by nausea and sensitivity to light and sound	A type of migraine headache that is typically more severe. Can be felt on both sides of the head.

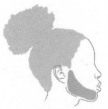 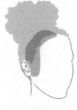 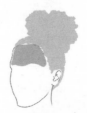 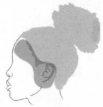

DENTAL	**NECK**	**TENSION**	**TMJ**
Pain is felt across upper and lower jaw. Can start near the ear and even travel down the neck.	Pain can be felt in most parts of the head but tends to be only on one side.	Usually affects both sides of the head either around the temples or across the forehead.	Pain aound the temple and in front of the ear. Can be on one or both sides.

TENSION HEADACHES

Selma worked as a teacher and was quite stressed with her job. Her posture was poor as she hunched over a computer in the evenings and her shoulders were rolled forwards. She came to me with tension headaches, and I massaged the back of her neck and head. She tried some exercises at home to open up her chest and her headaches went away.

The most common of all the headaches in Figure 4.1 is a *tension* headache, which is a general catch-all description for a classic headache and, as its name describes, links the headache to tension or muscle spasms in the neck, face, and head. This might not sound like good news to someone who is suffering from a tension headache, but when tense muscles are the potential root cause of a condition it means that a treatment can be provided. It's important to note that this type of headache has also been linked to stress, anxiety, and depression; and there is more about stress in Chapter 18.

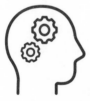

Start with your pain scale and **STOP**, and then consider if any of the following apply:

- **S**ite: Affects both sides of the head and sometimes the back of the head. Commonly felt across the forehead.

- **T**ype: A tight band of pain or pressure. It can be a mild to moderate dull ache. It won't pulse.

- **O**nset: It can be sudden or gradual, lasting from thirty minutes to a week. The pain can be constant during this length of time.

- **P**rovoked by: Stress, lack of sleep, missed meals, driving, posture-related issues from sitting, muscle tension in the neck and shoulders.

SELF HELP

- At home, try to reduce any immediate stress that you are feeling via breathing exercises or a change of environment. Drink water regularly throughout the day, try to get more sleep, or have a nap if you can. A cold compress can help as well.

- Keep a diary to help you recognize any potential triggers.

- You can self-massage the suboccipital muscles by lying on your back with a tennis or golf ball positioned underneath the base of your skull. Use your head to roll the ball around these muscles to relieve any tension there (see Figure 4.2).

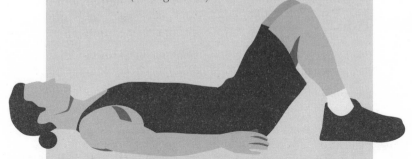

FIG. 4.2
SELF-MASSAGE OF
SUBOCCIPITAL MUSCLES

- You can see an osteopath or a chiropractor for this condition.

- A therapist should massage the muscles around the neck, shoulders, and back of the head, particularly the tiny suboccipital muscles at the base of the skull (see Figure 4.3), as they can contribute to tension headaches if they are tight.

- Gentle mobilization and clicking of the neck can also help relieve tension headaches. If a joint is slightly out of sync it means that the neck muscles will be overworked, which makes them tight, and this can impact on the muscles in the face and head.

- Gentle traction using the fingertips at the base of the skull and first vertebra is useful as it relieves the pressure on the joints in the neck. Dry needling the back of the neck can also help relieve tension in the neck muscles.

FIG. 4.3
SUBOCCIPITAL MUSCLES
AT BASE OF SKULL

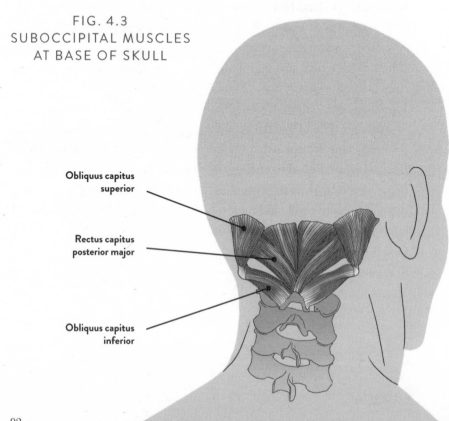

Obliquus capitus
superior

Rectus capitus
posterior major

Obliquus capitus
inferior

MIGRAINES

Becky had migraines twice a year, when she had to help organize large-scale events for work. These were her most stressful weeks of the year and the worst time for her to be incapacitated for a day or two. When I first met her, it was a month before the first event and together we devised a plan with the aim of preventing the migraines from happening. Becky increased her sleep and limited her screen time. I treated her every week and massaged her face, neck, shoulders, and the back of her head and used light traction on her neck. She managed to stay migraine-free throughout the entire event.

Migraines are the most common of the moderate to severe headaches. Despite around 10 per cent of the population suffering from them, their cause is still unknown. Women are three times more likely to suffer from migraines than men. The general theory is that migraines happen when there is a disruption in the chemicals, nerves, and blood vessels within the brain, resulting in a mixture of nerve and tissue pain. Around half of the people who suffer from migraines have a close relative who also has them, so genetics may play a role.

Some people have warning signs that a migraine is on its way, called *auras*, which are neurological signals such as flashing lights or spots in their vision. Others don't have any warning at all. The clients I normally see with migraines are female and can be of any age.

Another type of headache is a *hormonal* headache, which is similar to a migraine except it is usually on both sides of the head. These headaches are linked to changes in women's hormonal cycles and can be triggered by their menstrual cycle, the first trimester of pregnancy, the contraceptive pill, and menopause. Women with migraines should consider whether they might be hormonal headaches and look for any links with their menstrual cycle.

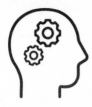

Start with your pain scale and **STOP**, and then consider if any of the following apply:

- **S**ite: Normally on one side of the face or head. Hormonal migraines might be on both sides of the face.

- **T**ype: Pulsing, throbbing. The pain can be mild to severe. There can be nausea and vomiting as well.

- **O**nset: Gradual. Some people can have several a week, whereas others might go years between migraines. They can last between four hours and three days.

- **P**rovoked by: Bright lights, loud noises, and bending forwards.

SELF HELP

- At home, try to lie down in a quiet, dark room. Place a cold compress or towel on your face and drink plenty of fluids.

- Keep a diary to help you recognize any potential triggers, particularly if you suspect they are hormonal migraines.

PROFESSIONAL HELP

- You can see a chiropractor or osteopath.

- A therapist should massage the muscles around the face, scalp, neck, shoulder, and jaw. When a client comes to me in the middle of a migraine, I will usually dry needle the neck and the trapezius muscle that stretches from the base of the skull, down through the neck.

- Gentle traction at the back of the neck between the skull and first vertebra is also beneficial for migraines.

SINUSITIS

The first time I heard about sinuses was when my older brother was 16 years old. His sinuses became blocked and the area above his eyes was very puffy. He was eventually given antibiotics, but this didn't seem to help. It became so bad that he was admitted to hospital for two weeks and had two operations to widen his nasal passages, but this didn't work either. He was told by his consultant to sniff salted water into his nose, and this was what eventually resolved the condition after a year.

The sinuses are four pairs of hollow spaces in our bones that connect with each other. They are about an inch long and situated around the face (see Figure 4.4). They are usually filled with air and lined with a thin tissue that produces mucus. If they are blocked then they can become inflamed, which often happens after a cold or flu. If you read Chapter 3, then you will know that the '–itis' suffix on a word indicates inflammation. Therefore, *sinusitis* is the inflammation of the sinuses. The maxillary sinus in the cheekbones is the largest of the sinuses and the most common sinus to become inflamed.

....

FIG. 4.4
LOCATION OF THE SINUSES

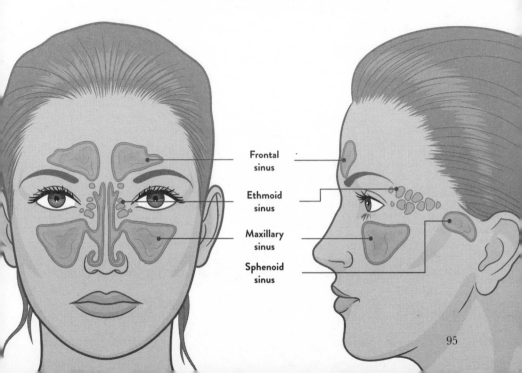

Frontal sinus

Ethmoid sinus

Maxillary sinus

Sphenoid sinus

Sinusitis can also result from allergies, as was the case with my brother. I asked him about this recently and he told me that he blames carnation flowers, as his condition started at school on Valentine's Day. He was a prefect at the time and had to hand out flowers to hundreds of pupils, but then his flower allergy irritated his sinuses and caused them to become inflamed. He won't go anywhere near carnations to this day.

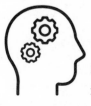 Start with your pain scale and **STOP**, and then consider if any of the following apply:

- **S**ite: This depends on which of the sinuses is blocked. Pain can be felt across the front of the face or only in specific areas. It can sometimes lead to pain in the teeth and ears.

- **T**ype: A dull pain with a feeling of pressure. There can also be swelling, a blocked or runny nose, a reduced sense of smell, difficulty breathing, fever, tiredness, or a cough. Parts of the face may be tender to touch.

- **O**nset: Sudden or gradual, lasting for a few days or several weeks.

- **P**rovoked: Often worse at night. If it's an allergic reaction, it can be provoked by dust, strong perfume, etc. – whatever is the root cause of the allergy.

SELF HELP

- At home you can use a nasal decongestant or saltwater nasal sprays.

- You can also try a self-drainage technique when lying down. Use two or three of your finger pads and tap below your eyes, between your eyes, on the cheek bones, and in front and behind the ears. Next, do small circular massages where the sinuses are located. Finish off with long sweeping strokes at the front of the neck, from the jaw line down to the collar bone.

- You can see an osteopath for the treatment of sinusitis. If the symptoms last more than ten days, you should see your doctor as you might need antibiotics or a steroid spray.

- Osteopaths treat sinusitis by using drainage techniques around the face, the front of the neck, and chest. In my experience this is effective, but should be accompanied by massage and possibly mobilization of the neck. I'd also massage all the way down to the shoulders and check if the lymph nodes in the armpits and neck are swollen.

TEMPOROMANDIBULAR JOINT (TMJ) DISORDER

The jaw is made up of two bones, called the *temporal* and the *mandible*, which form a joint. The mandible is the only bone in the face that visibly moves. It is also the strongest bone in the face (see Figure 4.5).

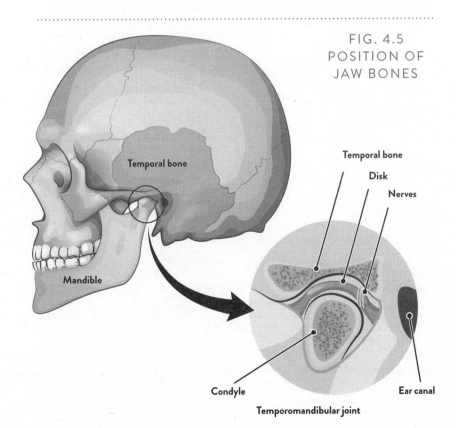

FIG. 4.5
POSITION OF
JAW BONES

Temporal bone

Mandible

Temporal bone

Disk

Nerves

Condyle

Ear canal

Temporomandibular joint

There can be many reasons why you have jaw pain: for example, dental issues, stress, clenching of the jaw, a misalignment of the jaw, direct trauma, or general wear and tear. Something as simple as clenching and grinding your teeth can lead to jaw pain. Also, increased tension in the muscles that help us chew can eventually lead to a stiff jaw, sore temples, headaches, jaw pain, and even ringing in the ears. If you have difficulties opening or closing your mouth, or any discomfort when using your jaw, it might be an early warning sign of an impending jaw condition.

The most common jaw condition I see is temporomandibular joint (TMJ) disorder, which is named after the joint in the jaw where pain can occur. In my experience, the pain around the jaw and ear is usually caused by the muscles surrounding the joint rather than the joint itself. TMJ problems can often arise if you clench or grind your jaw as this can affect the muscles used for chewing, and can overwork or strain them. The masseter muscle in the jaw is the strongest muscle in the body (see Figure 4.6).

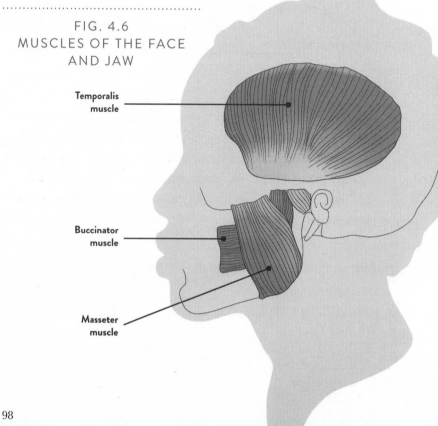

FIG. 4.6
MUSCLES OF THE FACE
AND JAW

Temporalis
muscle

Buccinator
muscle

Masseter
muscle

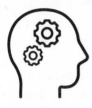

Start with your pain scale and **STOP**, and then consider if any of the following apply:

- **S**ite: Pain can be in or around the jaw, ears, or temples.

- **T**ype: It is either an intermittent dull ache or a sharp pain. It might also be tender to touch. There can also be clicking, cracking, locking, rubbing, or a catching sensation. You might also have earache.

- **O**nset: It can either be sudden or gradual.

- **P**rovoked by: Chewing, talking, smiling, trying to open the mouth fully, eating particularly hard food.

SELF HELP

- At home, you can apply ice to try and relieve any tenderness in the jaw. You should also try some of the self-massaging techniques below.

PROFESSIONAL HELP

- You can see an osteopath or chiropractor.

- A therapist should try to loosen up the tense muscles around the jaw, starting with the temporalis muscle that stretches across the side of the skull above the ear (see Figure 4.6). I've found the most effective way of massaging the muscles on the cheek near the jaw is to wear a surgical glove and put my thumb inside the client's mouth. I'll then pinch the client's mouth with my index finger on their outside cheek, as the client opens and closes their mouth. I also massage the muscles around the jaw from the inside of the client's mouth.

- Mobilization of the TMJ and cervical spine can also help release an out-of-sync joint. The vertebrae at the top of the spine can sometimes have an impact on the muscles around the jaw. If there is a large misalignment of the TMJ it will need to be clicked back into place, but this should only be done by a highly skilled therapist.

- Because the masseter muscle is so strong, it can often be too tender to touch. In this case, I would use dry needling or cold laser therapy first.

OTHER COMMON HEAD AND FACIAL CONDITIONS

- *Cluster headaches* are among the worst types of headaches. They're not as common as tension headaches and migraines, but are usually more severe than both of them. They affect one side of the face and usually centre around the eye. They are described as a sharp, burning, piercing sensation, and can be accompanied by a blocked nose and watery eyes. It is thought that they might be provoked by drinking alcohol or strong odours.

- *Trigeminal neuralgia* is one of the worst pains I have seen in my clients. It affects the trigeminal nerve in the lower part of the face. It is a very sudden, severe pain and is usually only on one side of the face.

MASSAGE FOR THE HEAD AND FACE

Our faces have forty-three muscles and, like the muscles in any other area of the body, they can become tight through overuse. Therefore, some light self-massage can help restore movement and alleviate tension in this often-overlooked area of the body. You don't even have to be in any pain or discomfort to benefit, as it will stimulate your face and, overall, you should feel more energized. Try as many of these massaging techniques as you want to and when you find one that helps your condition try to use it regularly.

- Starting at the outside of your nose, use circular massaging motions along the cheekbones to the sides of your head. Splay your fingers out to your scalp and lightly massage above the hairline.

- If the scalp muscles become tense, they can cause a tightness that can bring on a tension headache. To help prevent this, try to massage your scalp regularly. Splay your fingers out across your head and massage in small circles, using a firm pressure across your scalp. Concentrate on the area around your temples and the front and back of your ears.

- Hold the back of your head with your hands and place your thumbs underneath the bottom of your skull. Press your thumbs into the base of your skull and hold for five seconds. Alternate this with circular motions across your scalp with your finger pads.

- After washing your hands, place a clean finger inside your mouth to the side, right at the back. Use small circular motions to work your way around the muscles in front of the joint and down towards the bottom teeth (see Figure 4.7).

- After washing your hands, place a clean thumb on the inside of your mouth and press on the inside of your cheek. Gently push the cheek outwards and hold for five seconds (see Figure 4.8).

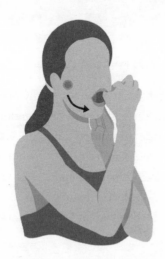

FIG. 4.7
MASSAGE THE MUSCLES
IN FRONT OF THE JOINT

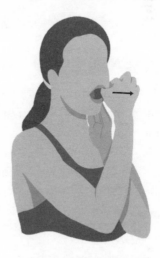

FIG. 4.8
MASSAGING BY PUSHING
THE CHEEK OUTWARDS

CHAPTER 5

Neck

How much time during the day do you spend looking down at your phone, desk, or laptop? Probably quite a lot. These adjustments we have made in our modern lives are not suited to a healthy neck and people often accept aches in this area as part of life. Our posture has become compromised, and we have forgotten what our necks were designed to do.

SYMPTOMS CHECK

IS YOUR NECK HEALTHY?

Try the following slowly, so you don't wrench any of your muscles. A healthy neck should be able to:

1
Turn to both sides so that you are looking towards where your shoulders are pointing. Your shoulders should remain completely still, as often people twist their back when doing this and think that they have full movement in their necks. Therefore, do this in front of a mirror or ask someone else to watch you.

2
Get your chin to your breastplate.

3
Roll your head back so your nose is nearly pointing to the sky. When you do this, you shouldn't feel any pain.

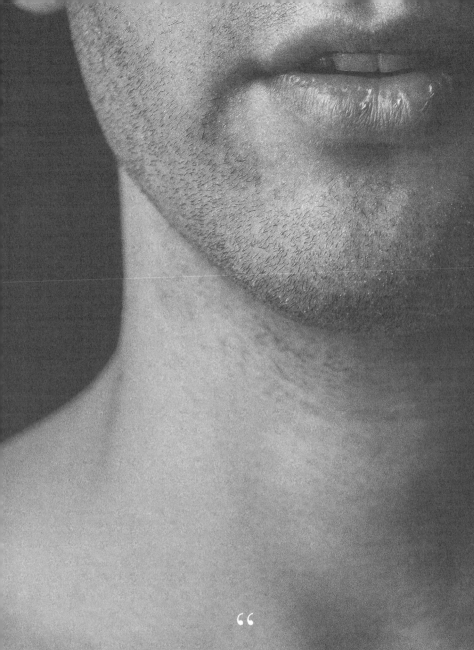

"

Our posture has become compromised,
and we have forgotten what our necks
were designed to do.

"

There are over twenty muscles in your neck used to support and move your head, but they also help with basic functions like breathing and swallowing. Most of the sensory organs are in our head, so it's important that our necks function fully so we can assess our surroundings – our early ancestors would have scanned the horizon regularly throughout their day in search of food, hunting opportunities, or to check for danger.

As you can see from Figure 5.1, the muscles in the neck stretch into other areas of the body, from the base of the skull to the shoulder blades and through to the back. The front of the neck is just as important as the back of the neck as there are postural muscles there as well. These muscles also benefit from exercises and massage and are often neglected.

FIG. 5.1
THE MUSCLES OF THE NECK

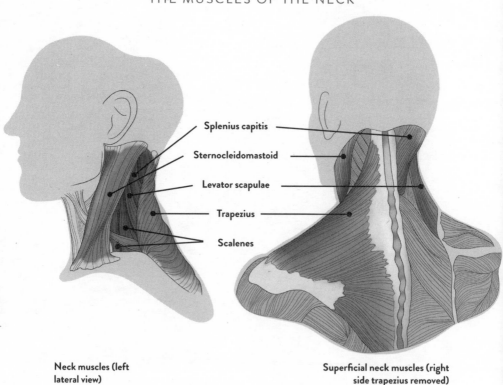

Splenius capitis
Sternocleidomastoid
Levator scapulae
Trapezius
Scalenes

Neck muscles (left lateral view)

Superficial neck muscles (right side trapezius removed)

Down the back of your spine are pairs of small joints called facets and there are seven sets of them in your neck. You therefore have fourteen of these joints in your neck alone. These joints have multiple functions, which includes movement in your spine. Most of the ability to rotate your neck is between the highest two, and if you lose the mobility there then it can affect everything lower down. Facet joints can become inflamed and stiff, even locking sometimes.

FIG. 5.2
CERVICAL SPINE

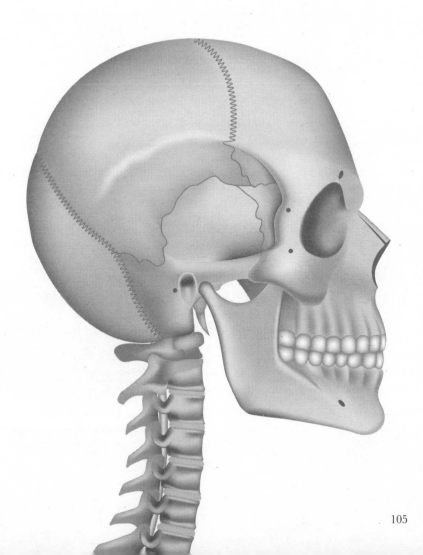

We should be aware of several warning flags when it comes to the neck, so always seek urgent medical attention if you experience any of the following: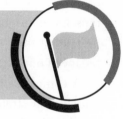

- Shooting pins and needles, tingling sensations, pain, or weakened grip in both arms
- Stiff neck with headache or fever
- If you've had a fall and are in constant pain
- Suffered trauma to the head or neck
- Been involved in a recent road-traffic accident and have neck pain
- Constant pain that nothing can lessen, including painkillers
- Have neck pain and a history of cancer
- A stiff neck and one of the worst headaches you have ever experienced
- Pain is a six or above out of ten on the pain scale
- Inability to sleep at all during the night
- Nausea or vomiting
- A new lump or swelling in the neck

MOST COMMON NECK CONDITIONS: STRAIN TO THE NECK MUSCLES

Let's start with the good news for necks – it's very rare that there is a muscle tear. If you are feeling the type of pain that suggests tissue damage, such as sharp twinges, aching, or throbbing then it is much more likely to be a strained muscle than a tear. This is often caused by a shortened muscle or overworked muscle due to your posture. If you think back to the case of the tiler in Chapter 2, there was no balance in his movements; he constantly leaned to his left and so, his muscles became shortened. If you are always looking down, the muscles at the back of your neck are lengthened and the scalene muscles at the front of your neck are shortened, so they need to be balanced out through stretches.

A common muscle to strain in your neck is the trapezius, a large muscle that stretches from the base of your skull through to your shoulder blades and down the back (see Figure 5.1). Another is the levator scapulae that attaches to the top of the cervical spine down to the shoulder blade. Both muscles are used a lot, so they become overworked and are consequently strained.

There are also many ligaments in the neck so it might be that you have sprained one of these. The treatment for them is similar to that for a muscle strain.

Keep in mind that a strain to the neck can be as simple as a mild ache or a feeling that 'something isn't quite right', all the way through to extremely limited movement on both sides of the neck. If you've had the condition for over three months then it is chronic, and you should seek medical advice even if the strain is mild.

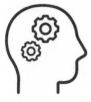

Start with your pain scale and **STOP**, and then consider the following:

- **S**ite: The pain will be fixed and more commonly felt unilaterally; that is, only on one side of the neck.

- **T**ype: It's often a twinging pain when moving the head towards the shoulder, or a dull ache or stiffness in any part of the neck. The pain can feel deep or superficial depending on which muscle it is.

- **O**nset: A strain is typically gradual and builds over days or weeks.

- **P**rovoked: Moving the head to the side often provokes the pain. You also need to think about your posture. Are you sitting at a desk or in front of a computer for hours every day? And is it worse when you do this?

CHECK YOUR NECK

- If you have difficulty turning your head, ask someone to place the pad of their thumb at the back of your neck, right next to your spine, and press down with a mild to moderate pressure. Then slowly try to move your head left or right ten times. If that makes it better, then it is a good sign that it's a moderate strain and not anything more serious.

- If you look down and there is pain in your mid-back or shoulder, it might be a strain to the trapezius, which is a muscle that covers the shoulders, neck, and upper back.

- If applying something warm to the neck helps alleviate the pain, it's a good sign it is a muscle strain and not an inflamed disc bulge.

- If you have lost any power in your upper limbs, or don't have a full range of movement in either shoulder, this would suggest a nerve-root irritation or a referred pain from a joint, which both rule out a strain.

MYTH BUSTERS

Many people have massage guns, which can be beneficial when used properly, but so many of us don't do this. Massage guns aren't designed to be used on all parts of the body, despite what the labels say. I wouldn't ever recommend using a massage gun directly on the neck as the vibration rattles through your head, which isn't very relaxing. Instead, use it on the muscles around the top of your back.

PROFESSIONAL HELP

- For a general neck strain, you should see an osteopath, physiotherapist or chiropractor. For a milder neck strain, you could also see a skilled massage therapist.

- A therapist should check the range of movement in your neck, shoulders, and mid-back. The last is very important as a lack of full movement in the mid-back can cause a strain in your neck. The therapist should also lightly massage and loosen up the muscles all around your neck, not just the one where you are feeling pain. The muscles at the front of the neck should also be treated as these are often overlooked.

- Throughout the process the therapist should concentrate on the mobilization of the neck instead of clicking it. Clicking might be necessary if it appears that there is an underlying joint issue as well, but this should only be done after mobilization and massage, rather than right at the beginning of the session.

- Dry needling can help if someone has a severe strain and is sensitive to touch. Afterwards, they will usually be less tender.

- If the strain is very acute, then cold laser therapy can help.

Sleeping badly is one of the most common causes of both muscle strains and joint issues in the neck. This is particularly common in people who sleep on their fronts. If you sleep on your front, turning your head to the side on your pillow will shorten one side of your neck muscles and lengthen the others, potentially leading to muscle strain.

Joint issues often happen when people have the wrong type of pillows or mattresses, and are common in people who travel for work as they're always changing beds and pillows. It is quite common for people to wake up and find their necks are locked.

There is more about sleep in Chapter 19.

JOINT CONDITIONS

PATIENT FILES: JOINT CONDITIONS

My client, Rosa, woke up one morning and couldn't turn her neck to the side to turn her alarm off. I saw her later in the afternoon and she had to turn her whole body to the right to look in that direction. She thought she'd trapped a nerve, but it was clearly a joint issue brought on by the way she had slept the previous night. I mobilized her neck joint back into place, and so returned the full range of movement that she had been missing.

Our bodies have 360 joints. Fourteen of the smaller ones, called the facet joints, are in the neck and they help us look to the side, up and down, and rotate the neck. They were not designed to cope with some of the demands of modern life and therefore can lock up, sometimes without us even knowing about it.

If a joint locks, then it doesn't always mean an extreme inability to move our neck, like in Rosa's case. Even if we feel no pain when our joints lock, our muscles will still try to overcompensate and this causes them to become strained.

When someone is unable to move their neck from one side to the other it can be a severe strain, but it's more likely to be a facet lock or dysfunction to the facets. The first two facets allow most of the rotation in the neck and if they lock up, then the lower ones take on more of this responsibility. People spend years without knowing they have a locked facet because they might not be in pain. However, most people with this condition will feel some degree of pain around the neck.

A facet lock can happen by itself or can involve a nerve as well. If you feel classic nerve pain, such as possible referred pain, shooting pain, tingling, burning, numbness, or pins and needles, along with a lack of mobility, then it might be that the joint has pinched a nerve. In this case, you should book an appointment with your doctor for medication, and an osteopath or chiropractor for treatment.

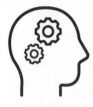 Start with your pain scale and **STOP**, and then consider the following:

- **S**ite: The pain is normally felt in the neck, but often not at the exact site of the joint that has a problem. It is common for there to be a referred pain either higher up or lower down in the neck than the actual joint that has been affected.

- **T**ype: Joint pain is usually described as a deep or dull ache, although it can sometimes be a sharp momentary pain when moved. It's possible there will be no pain at all, just a stiffness in the neck or lack of mobility. If it is acute, and only happened in the last few days, there may also be inflammation, so consider whether it is warm, red, or swollen. If it involves a nerve as well, there will also be shooting pains, tingling sensations, burning, and so on.

- **O**nset: It can be acute or chronic depending on when it began, and can also be a sudden or gradual pain. Usually, it will get worse if left untreated. Think about whether you woke up with it, as it's quite common for the joint to lock during sleep.

- **P**rovoked: The mobility exercises underneath the magnifying glass below should provide a good indication of whether it is a joint issue. A classic sign of a joint condition is that it hurts when you look up.

MORE USEFUL NECK CHECKS

- Check which movements are affected by going through the above symptoms check, as being unable to complete all these movements is a sign of a mobility issue with the neck.

- If a facet is locked there is normally difficulty with rolling your head directly back and then, still in this position, rotating your neck so you are looking slightly to the side, but with your nose still pointing upwards. It's really important when doing this to only hold the position for a second, as it's also a test for a functioning artery and shouldn't be held for long. If something feels wrong when you have done this test it might be a joint issue.

- Another check is to tilt your head to the side and then rotate it so you're trying to look at your shoulder. If something feels wrong, it might also be a joint issue.

SELF-HELP

At home, you can use several self-massage techniques. My favourite is to place my finger pads, with my fingers close together, on the bony prominence at the base of the back of my neck, or to the side of it, depending on where the pain is. Keep your elbow up so it is facing forwards and then gently drop your elbow. Your fingers will naturally follow and pull down the side of your neck. You can do this with both hands if the pain is on both sides or even use a crossover. So, with your left hand place your finger pads to the right of the spine, and vice versa. Even small circular massages over the spine are beneficial.

- If you suspect a joint condition then you should see an osteopath, chiropractor, or physiotherapist. You could also see a massage therapist who is skilled in soft tissue and mobilization of this specific area.

- It's important that if you see a therapist they don't start by clicking your neck. They should begin firstly by treating the tissue surrounding the joint through massage and mobilization. The joint might even go back into place through mobilization alone, without the need for clicking. Clicking should be the last thing they try, and only if necessary.

- Dry needling can also help treat the surrounding tissue if the muscles are too tender to touch, as just a few needles are needed around the joint in question.

- Gentle traction of the area by the therapist can help as well, as this helps alleviate the pressure on the joint. Traction is a separation of the vertebrae by pulling at your neck in a specific way.

- If a facet joint does have to be clicked back into place, you will normally only need to do this on one joint. Your neck is not a piano – all the keys don't need to be tuned. In most cases, the therapist will also need to treat the tissues around the joint to help stabilize it and prevent the same condition from recurring. If you've had your neck clicked back into place, don't apply heat as it's already warm. The best thing you can do is apply ice. There's more information about clicking in Chapter 16.

PATIENT FILES: DISC BULGES AND NERVE-ROOT IRRITATION

Miriam came to see me because of a loss of grip in one of her hands and shooting pain down her shoulder. When I examined her, I was more interested in her neck than her hand. Thirty years of working at a desk had changed her posture, so her shoulders were rounded and her neck hunched forwards. It was here that a nerve had been trapped, causing the pain and loss of grip in her hand and, with some gentle mobilization, it was freed.

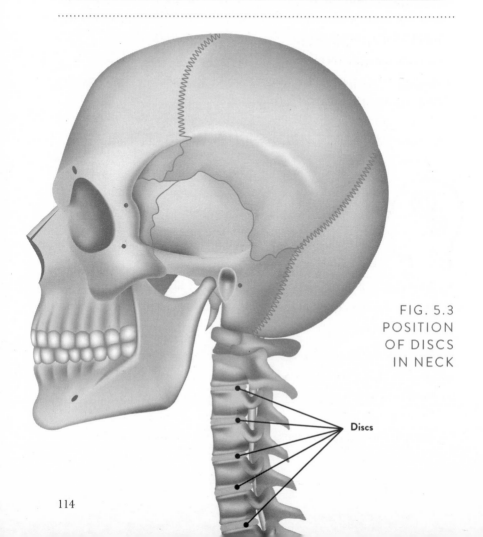

FIG. 5.3
POSITION
OF DISCS
IN NECK

Discs

We couldn't have a section on the neck without looking at nerves as well. The most common type of nerve condition in the neck is when one of the six discs presses on a nerve. This is what had happened to Miriam. This happens when the disc bulges because of trauma or, more commonly, as the result of a loss of height between the discs as we age.

Disc bulges are more common in the lower back as there is more weight pushing down on them there. However, they are still relatively common in the neck, but this usually happens because of bad posture and poor muscle condition, as in Miriam's case. These can both cause problems with the discs, because your muscles act partially as shock absorbers and if they are tight then they are not as efficient.

There are two different types of disc bulges. A *central* disc bulge is when it presses on the spinal cord and symptoms of nerve pain are felt in *both* arms. This is one of the warning signs listed under the flag symbol at the beginning of the chapter (page 106) and you should seek immediate medical attention. More commonly, the disc bulge is *to one side*, so one part of the disc presses on a nerve root, which causes similar symptoms but only down one arm.

You can have a disc bulge without nerve-root irritation but if left unchecked, it will usually result in it pressing on a nerve as the condition worsens.

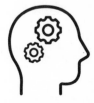 Start with your pain scale and **STOP**, and then consider the following:

- **S**ite: Pain will be around the neck but there will normally be referred pain in the shoulders, arms, or hands. If there isn't any nerve-root irritation yet, it will be a localized pain around the disc in question.

- **T**ype: A disc bulge that has also irritated a nerve is normally described as a shooting pain down an arm, with tingling and weakness which can be felt in the shoulder, down the arm and in the hands and fingers.. It is usually a severe pain that people compare to a stabbing sensation or electrical shock. If the nerve hasn't been irritated yet, it will be a dull ache.

- **O**nset: Pain from a disc bulge is normally gradual as the disc slowly deteriorates. It can be sudden, but this is normally when trauma is involved, following a fall or car accident.

- **P**rovoked: If the pain increases when you cough and sneeze, it is likely to be a disc bulge as you will be more sensitive to the force travelling through the spine. Clients have told me they become scared of coughing and sneezing.

If there is pain in your neck when you look down, it is more likely that it's a disc issue rather than a joint problem.

If, when you move your neck, you feel a referred pain in your shoulder, mid-back or arm it's likely to be a nerve-root irritation in the neck.

WHERE IS THE SOURCE OF YOUR NECK CONDITION?

If you want to try and narrow down which level of the spine you are having a problem with, and it involves a nerve, first try and locate the area on your neck that is tender to touch. There are eight pairs of spinal nerves that run from C1 to T1 that can help you decide which of the seven vertebrae in the neck is affected. If you are also having difficulty with the following then it could be that you have a problem with a nerve at the level of a cervical vertebra, which can be confirmed by a scan. A sign of which level might be affected is when you experience a weakness in one of the following movements:

- C4: you have lost power when shrugging your shoulders

- C5: moving the arms away from the side of the body

- C6: bending your elbow so your arm comes towards your body or bending your wrist upwards

- C7: using your elbow to make your arm straight or bending your wrist down

- C8: moving your thumb away from your fingers

If you notice any weakness when you do the above movements, please let your doctor know.

OTHER COMMON NECK CONDITIONS

- If you are suffering from stress and anxiety, you can often get aches or tightness around your throat (see Chapter 18).

- Difficulties breathing or swallowing may be because of overuse of the scalene muscles at the front of the neck. Massage can help with this.

- Overuse of the muscles around the voice box can benefit from massage around the front of the neck. This is particularly common in singers.

- Cervical spondylosis is a degenerative condition where, over time, the discs in the neck become dehydrated and shrink. This is usually symptomless, but can cause the nerves to become pinched in the spinal cord.

- Osteophytes are bony lumps that grow on the spine or joints, usually in the neck. These can irritate a nerve by pressing on it.

SELF-HELP

- You can buy a traction machine to use at home. These can work well, but you should only buy one if a disc bulge has been diagnosed by a medical professional.

- You can perform light traction movements at home using a bath towel. Place the towel around the back of your neck so it hangs over both of your shoulders. Take each end of the towel in your hands and tilt your head downwards. Gently pull on both ends of the towel so that your arms are straight and point diagonally upwards. You should be making an upwards V shape with your arms.

- If you suspect that you have a disc bulge, then you should make an appointment with your doctor as you may need prescription painkillers and an X-ray or MRI scan.

- You can go to an osteopath, chiropractor, or physiotherapist for treatment.

- The best treatment for a disc bulge is traction as this separates the vertebrae, taking the pressure away from any nerves involved as well.

STRETCHES AND EXERCISES FOR THE NECK

Below are my favourite stretches and exercises that I recommend to all my clients with neck problems. They should be done slowly in smooth and gentle movements. If any of these make your condition worse, or are very painful, then you should stop immediately.

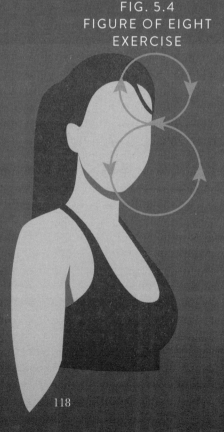

FIG. 5.4
FIGURE OF EIGHT
EXERCISE

1

It may sound a bit weird, but imagine you have two pencils where your eyes are and start drawing a figure of eight with your eyes (see Figure 5.4). As your neck loosens, make the 'eight' larger, but still within a comfortable range of movement. Draw this in both directions. After you have done this a few times, imagine the pencil is where your nose is and repeat the process again. Finally, place your imaginary pencil where your chin is and draw a few more. Moving the point of focus down through these positions helps loosen the muscles in the top, mid-area, and base of the neck. If you hear a few crackles when doing this, it's not something to worry about.

FIG. 5.5
CHIN TO COLLARBONE
EXERCISE

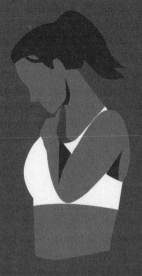
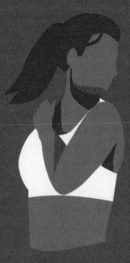

2

Place two fingers of your right hand just above the left side of your left collarbone and move your chin down to your fingers (see Figure 5.5). Then slowly move your head up and in the opposite direction away from your fingers. Repeat on both sides of your neck.

3

A good exercise for your neck is a simple one where you sit with your head facing forward and your shoulders are relaxed. Simply turn your head from side to side so you are looking towards each of your shoulders.

4

If you have a tennis ball, stand up against a wall and place the ball between the back of your neck and the wall. The ball should be pressed against your muscles on either side of your spine rather than directly on the spine. Using your neck to manoeuvre the ball, begin to roll it gently over the muscles on either side of your spine. You can also do this exercise lying on the floor.

5

Poor posture makes your shoulders roll in, which pulls your neck forward. Begin to start opening up your chest by holding your arms straight at a ten and two position on a clock. Hold this position with a relaxed neck and gently draw your arms back by squeezing your shoulder blades together.

CHAPTER 6

Shoulders

Our shoulders have a huge range of movement but the downside to this is instability, and therefore vulnerability. Consequently, shoulder problems are very common. This is partly because the shoulder is one of the most complex joints in the body: it isn't just one joint, it's four (see Figure 6.1). These four mobile connectors allow the shoulder to have a wide range of movement that perhaps a lot of us take for granted. We can rotate our arms in wide circles both backwards and forwards, and lift our arms up towards the sky – imagine trying to do all of that with your hips.

These joints need lots of ligaments to keep them in place and the ligaments in the shoulder are notoriously weak compared to the ones in the hip. This means the muscles in the shoulder often have to take on the added role of stabilizing the shoulder joints, which overworks them and causes wear and tear.

> The shoulder is one of the most complex joints of the body.

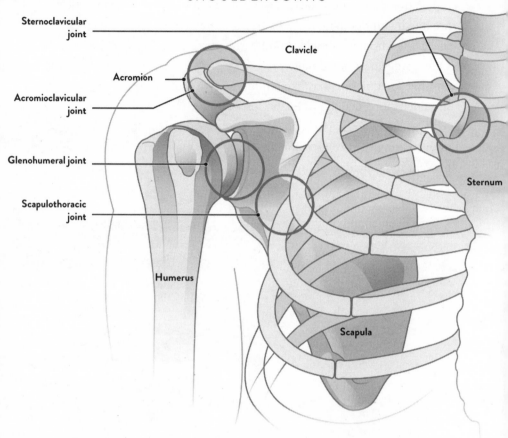

FIG. 6.1
SHOULDER JOINTS

Sternoclavicular joint

Acromion

Acromioclavicular joint

Glenohumeral joint

Scapulothoracic joint

Humerus

Clavicle

Sternum

Scapula

Just to raise your arm away from your body involves several different sets of muscles and joints, and even your collarbone has to rotate. All it takes is for one muscle to become strained, not work well, and then the other muscles try to compensate, which can lead to a muscle, tendon, or ligament tear. It's a domino effect and because there are so many parts involved in the shoulder's movement, it can often be difficult to pinpoint the root cause of the problem.

In my experience the most common cause of shoulder injuries are poor posture, when the shoulders are rolled inwards, or repetitive actions that cause wear and tear. If your job demands that you have to repeat the same action constantly, think about how well your shoulders are moving. It doesn't have to be heavy manual work – I've seen plenty of clients who have shoulder problems from using a computer mouse. Often, we expect our shoulder to compensate for lack of movement in another area; if our wrist is painful then we often begin to move our shoulder more, leading to further problems.

The shoulder is particularly vulnerable to recurring injuries, so after treating the problem you should begin strengthening exercises to prevent it happening again.

ARE YOUR SHOULDERS HEALTHY?

SYMPTOMS
CHECK

Healthy shoulders should be able to do the following:

- Keeping your arm straight, lift it away from your body in a semicircle until your hand points upwards. Check this in a mirror or ask someone to watch you as it's common to drop your other shoulder if there is an impairment.

- Keep your arm straight then lift it forwards in a semicircle until your fingers point upwards.

- Move your hand behind your back until you touch the bottom of your opposite shoulder blade from below.

- Check in a mirror whether your shoulders roll in. Also check for asymmetries. You might have a dominant shoulder that is lower than the other and will have more muscle bulk.

- Move your arm across your body and touch the outside of the opposite shoulder.

- Complete circular arm swings both forwards and backwards.

The most commonly injured muscles and tendons in the shoulder are a set of four called the rotator cuff muscles (see Figure 6.2). Each of these plays an individual role in stabilizing the shoulder and its movement. Have a look at Chapter 3 if you think you might have a shoulder strain or tear, and for guidance on how to tell the difference between the two.

FIG. 6.2
ROTATOR CUFF MUSCLES

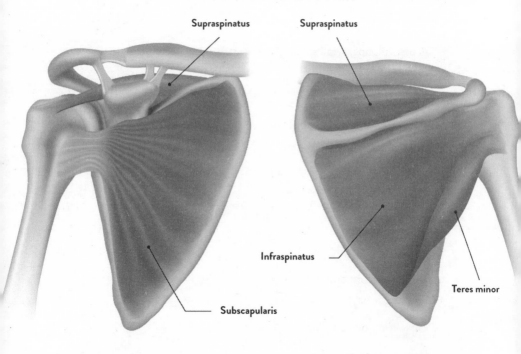

Supraspinatus   Supraspinatus

Infraspinatus

Teres minor

Subscapularis

FRONT VIEW   **BACK VIEW**

When thinking about the shoulder always consider referred pain. Could the source of pain be from your neck? If it feels like a nerve-type pain or is across the muscles at the top of your back, then it might be a referred pain from the neck and you should read that chapter.

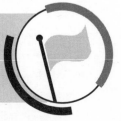

There are several warning flags when it comes to the shoulder, so always seek urgent medical attention if you experience any of the following:

- A painful, hot, swollen joint that you are unable to move

- Near-complete loss of movement in an arm and the urge to cradle it to hold it in place

- Pain and weakness in both shoulders and a headache on both sides of your head

- Constant pain after a fall or trauma to the shoulder

- The suspicion that you may have dislocated or fractured your shoulder

- Shoulder pain and a history of cancer

- Tenderness on any of the bones in the shoulder and they are swollen or have changed shape

- New lump or bump on any aspect of the shoulder

- Pain at eight or above out of ten on the pain scale

- Inability to sleep at all during the night

MOST COMMON SHOULDER CONDITIONS: IMPINGEMENT

The first thing to say about a shoulder impingement is that it is incredibly common – it's estimated that one in five people will suffer a shoulder impingement at some point in their life (see Figure 6.3). It happens when one of the tendons in your rotator cuff, or a bursa, gets trapped or caught, or rubs in the space just below your shoulder blade. Alternatively, there can be a bony growth that catches against the rotator cuff.

Impingements are common, as they usually occur because of poor posture, degeneration, overuse, general wear and tear, and repetitive movements – basically, from using your shoulder a lot over several years. This problem is more common in people over the age of 35, as it is often linked to overuse of the muscles, but can happen at any age.

PATIENT FILES: IMPINGEMENT

George was 42 years old when he came to see me. In the space of a couple of months he had gone from someone who enjoyed playing golf every weekend to not being able to put on his shirt. He was really worried that this was the beginning of a debilitating illness and was surprised when I asked if I could take a few photos of him from the side and back. I showed him my screen and he was able to see that his shoulders were rounded in the side shot and that his shoulder blade drifted to the right – it was very clear from the images, but he'd never been able to see himself from that angle before.

He worked in an office and sat at a desk for eight hours a day and consequently had poor posture. I treated the stiffened muscles around his shoulders and together we came up with some stretches he could do at work. He took them seriously and did them regularly throughout the day, usually when he was thinking about how to respond to an email. In a week he had less pain and could do up his shirt by himself. A few weeks after that he was back happily playing golf.

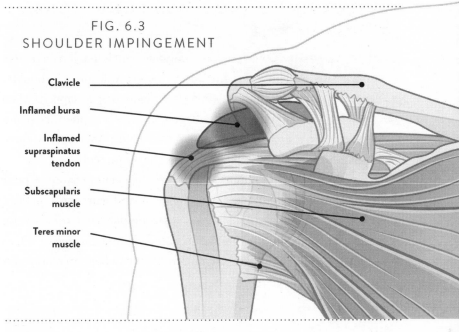

FIG. 6.3
SHOULDER IMPINGEMENT

Clavicle

Inflamed bursa

Inflamed
supraspinatus
tendon

Subscapularis
muscle

Teres minor
muscle

Start with your pain scale and **STOP**, and then consider the following:

- **S**ite: Pain is usually felt around the top or the outer side of the shoulder.

- **T**ype: It is usually a dull, aching pain that is present even when you're not using your arm. There is often a weakness or sharp pain when lifting your arm or reaching for things. It is common for the pain to disrupt sleep.

- **O**nset: It's most common for it to come on gradually over weeks or months. It can start suddenly, particularly if you've fallen with an outstretched arm.

- **P**rovoked: Pain increases when you lift or lower the arm, especially over the head. Everyday activities such as combing your hair, brushing your teeth, reaching for a plate in a cupboard, or getting dressed are often affected.

FIG. 6.4
HOW TO CHECK FOR SHOULDER IMPINGEMENT

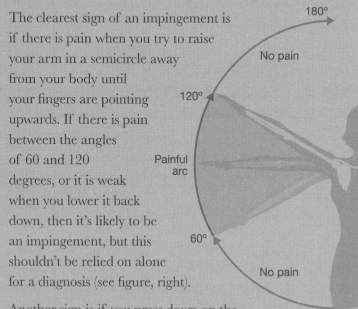

- The clearest sign of an impingement is if there is pain when you try to raise your arm in a semicircle away from your body until your fingers are pointing upwards. If there is pain between the angles of 60 and 120 degrees, or it is weak when you lower it back down, then it's likely to be an impingement, but this shouldn't be relied on alone for a diagnosis (see figure, right).

180°

No pain

120°

Painful arc

60°

No pain

- Another sign is if you press down on the supraspinatus with your fingers and try and raise your arm in the same way as indicated in the point above. If the movement is less painful then this can be an indication of a shoulder impingement. The muscle works better because the pressure from your fingers helps remove the pressure from the trapped tendon.

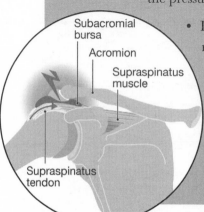

Subacromial bursa

Acromion

Supraspinatus muscle

Supraspinatus tendon

- If you are not sure whether you have rounded shoulders, try to retract them (this is the opposite of rolling them forwards) and see if you can lift your arm higher. If you can, it shows that your shoulders are rounded and you need to do some exercises to open up your chest.

SELF-HELP

- In the recovery period, it's best to keep the shoulder moving instead of resting it. If your pain is below level three and you are still able to move your shoulder, then avoid using a sling as this will only shorten and lengthen the muscles, and it will make it harder to achieve a full recovery. Instead, try to avoid movements that are sharp and very uncomfortable.

- After the pain has gone, strengthening exercises will be needed to improve the muscles surrounding the shoulder or the condition is likely to come back again.

- If you have rounded shoulders, then exercises to open up the chest will help.

PROFESSIONAL HELP

- With a suspected impingement, either a physiotherapist, osteopath or chiropractor should be the first line of call to confirm the diagnosis.

- A therapist should treat all four joints, as well as the rotator cuff muscles in the shoulder through massage and rhythmical, circling movements, in which their hands act to support the muscles. The aim is to loosen up the overworked muscle to take the pressure off the tendon. Shoulders are complex so it is always best to treat all the muscles. A good position to do this from is when the patient is lying on their side. Ideally, the neck, pectoral muscles, and ribs should be treated as well. The ribs are important because if they are tight, then they can clamp down on the shoulder blade.

- A doctor can give you a steroid injection if the pain doesn't go away.

It's often said that heat is better for shoulder pain than ice because ice 'freezes' the shoulder. This isn't true and the shoulder should be treated like any other part of the body: ice if there is inflammation; and contrast bathing, where you switch between heat and ice, if there is no inflammation.

INSTABILITY

PATIENT FILES: INSTABILITY

Sara had done gymnastics when she was younger, which had weakened her shoulder joint, so it felt 'loose'. After some treatment, she needed to build up the strength in her muscles and surrounding tissues to prevent the next dislocation being a full one.

We've probably all heard of shoulders being dislocated, but instability also covers the less extreme version when the ball joint moves out of the shallow socket by a small amount. Clients with a partial dislocation often refer to their shoulder as feeling 'loose', which is how Sara had described her shoulder to me when she first came to see me.

These smaller dislocations need to be dealt with quickly as they put a huge amount of stress on the surrounding tissues, wear them down, can result in a full dislocation (which is a warning flag and needs urgent medical attention at A&E), or a tear to the rotator cuff muscles.

A partial dislocation can either be when the ball joint pops out slightly and stays there, or, more commonly, when it returns to the socket by itself. This happens because the ligaments around the joint have been weakened, either because of repetitive movements or even just because the person was born that way. The tissue around the joint can be stretched or torn during a partial dislocation, and therefore, it's very likely to happen again.

If you have a fully dislocated shoulder, you will certainly know about it as you won't be able to move your arm and it will be extremely painful. It's also likely to happen because of trauma such as a fall.

Because it's such an obvious injury, the diagnosis sections below are for the subtler issue of a partial dislocation.

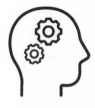

Start with your pain scale and **STOP**, and then consider the following:

- **S**ite: Pain is generally felt over the joint, especially at the front.

- **T**ype: It will probably be a sharp pain when it happens, but the shoulder will also feel loose, or as if it is giving away, or there may be swelling. There may also be pins and needles or numbness down the arm if there is also nerve damage.

- **O**nset: It is more likely to be a repetitive injury, although it can happen suddenly because of trauma.

- **P**rovoked: You will notice that you don't have a full range of movement and that some simple, everyday activities will provoke the shoulder into moving out of place.

There may be a clicking or a catching sensation when moving the arm.

A feeling of 'looseness' is often described, and is what sets instability apart from an impingement.

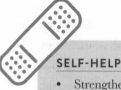

- Strengthening exercises for the muscles surrounding the shoulder are important because if you have instability, then the joint is going to keep on popping out until those muscles are strengthened and can hold it in place. You can either see a skilled therapist, who can work out a rehabilitation plan or, if you can't afford this, try the strengthening exercises at the end of this chapter.

PROFESSIONAL HELP

- If the shoulder has become fully dislocated, then you should immediately go to A&E for it to be manipulated back into place. You should never try to do this by yourself as it can damage the joint or tear the muscles surrounding it. Afterwards it will be very inflamed, so you should use **R**est, **I**ce, **C**ompression, and **E**levation (see page 70).

- If there is a partial dislocation then you can see a physiotherapist, osteopath, or chiropractor for treatment. They will put the joint back into place with gentle mobilization. The therapist should then look for the cause of why the joint has weakened and create an exercise plan to strengthen the area.

ARTHRITIS

PATIENT FILES: ARTHRITIS

Simon had played rugby in his younger days and was now in his sixties. His shoulder had been aching for years and there was clear instability there, which is common in people who have played rugby because it's a contact sport. The pain had increased in the previous couple of months and was now stopping him from lying on his side in bed. He'd also lost mobility in the shoulder as well. Unfortunately, the long-term stress on his shoulder joint had led to osteoarthritis. I first of all tried to reduce his pain with massage, and then increased his mobility with mobilization of the shoulder and surrounding joints.

Often when we think of arthritis we think of the hands or the knees, but arthritis in the shoulder is also incredibly common. A staggering one in three people over the age of 60 has some degree of shoulder arthritis. Arthritis is most common in people over the age of 50, but it can affect children and teenagers as well, particularly following an injury. There is more about osteoarthritis and rheumatoid arthritis in Chapter 3.

Osteoarthritis might be what you are heading for if you've had regular problems with your shoulder, such as an impingement or instability – there should be a large arrow pointing at osteoarthritis from the sections above (on Impingement and Instability), if these two conditions have been left untreated. This is exactly what had happened to Simon.

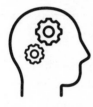 Start with your pain scale and **STOP**, and then consider the following:

- **S**ite: The pain can be in any part of the shoulder, either at the front or back, and can spread to the upper arm. If the pain is severe, it can radiate down the arm to the elbow and wrist.

- **T**ype: Arthritis feels like a deep ache. The key with arthritis is that you will feel stiffness in the affected area.

- **O**nset: The onset of the pain will be gradual, as will loss of movement in the shoulder.

- **P**rovoked: Changes in the weather can provoke the pain, as can lifting or carrying heavy objects. The pain is often worse in the mornings.

 A classic sign of arthritis is that you will be able to hear a creaking or clicking sound in your shoulder joints.

PROFESSIONAL HELP

- You can see an osteopath, physiotherapist or chiropractor for arthritis. Mobilization of the joint and hands-on work on the muscles and ligaments is key.

- In my experience, cold laser therapy works really well for arthritis in the shoulder.

MYTH BUSTERS

Arthritis can be a debilitating disease and often our instinct is to try and protect ourselves from movement. This is actually the opposite of what we should be doing as, without regular exercise and stretches, any remaining movement will reduce.

OTHER COMMON SHOULDER CONDITIONS

- A frozen shoulder is when abnormal bands of tissue grow in the joint and stiffen it. This is a complex condition that has three stages to it: freezing, frozen, and thawing out, and each one requires different treatment.

- Polymyalgia rheumatica is an inflammatory disorder that causes muscle stiffness and pain. It's more common in women and the pain will be in both shoulders. It is treated with steroids. It can be linked to inflammation around the arteries in the temples, so you should contact your doctor if you suspect you might have this condition.

- Bicep tendonitis is an inflammation of the upper bicep tendon that is attached to the shoulder joint. Common symptoms are pain in the front of the shoulder and weakness.

STRETCHES AND EXERCISES FOR SHOULDERS

The shoulder is a complex joint, but the best exercises and stretches for the above conditions are all the same. You should start with trying to correct your posture as this is often the root cause of shoulder problems. An experienced therapist or good personal trainer will help you devise a rehabilitation plan if you can afford this. As with all the exercises in the book, if they are painful or make your shoulder injury worse, then please stop them immediately.

FIG. 6.5

EXERCISES WITH RESISTANCE BAND

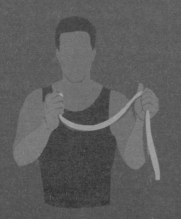 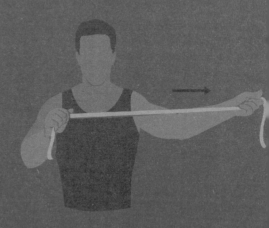

1

Many of the problems with shoulders comes from poor posture leading to rounded shoulders. To combat this, we need to do the opposite and open up our chests. Take each end of a bath towel in your hands and hold your arms high as if in a ten to two position on a clock, keeping your head facing forwards. It seems simple but the towel creates an extra level of resistance, and this exercise is very good for balancing out those rounded postures.

2

Another useful opening exercise is when you stand upright and grasp the wrist on your painful arm with the hand of your non-painful arm behind your back. Gently pull the painful arm away from your back until you feel a nice stretch in the painful shoulder. Hold it for a few seconds before releasing. Repeat this several times.

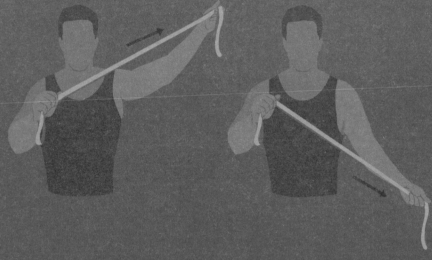

3

We've talked about how important
it is to strengthen the muscles in
the shoulder to prevent recurring
injuries. The best thing to use for
this is a resistance band, which is
like a large elastic band that provides
resistance when you exercise.
Holding one end of the band in
each hand, pull it outwards gently so
that you can feel the stretch on both
sides. In the same position, you can
also move just one arm upwards on
the outside of your body, so it is level
with your ear to work a different
set of muscles, like in the above
illustration.

4

Self-massage is really helpful for
shoulder injuries. If you have a
massage gun it is very effective to
use it on the front, side, and back
of the shoulder. If you don't have
one, then use the four fingertips of
the opposite arm on the front of the
shoulder and hold for five seconds
or make circular motions over your
clothes or with a bit of oil or cream.
The pressure from a tennis ball can
also be used.

CHAPTER 7

Upper back

L et's begin with where the upper back is. The easiest way to identify the upper back is to section off the middle part of the spine, which is called the *thoracic* spine (see Figure 7.1). It's the longest part of the spine and also the least mobile, so there are fewer disc problems here. The main job of the thoracic spine is to hold the ribs in place; these protect the heart and lungs. As you'll see from Figure 7.1, the area around the thoracic spine includes the ribs, the area between the shoulder blades, and the very bottom of the neck.

The upper back is the site of a lot of referred pain so it's always good to think about whether the source of the pain might be somewhere else (see Figure 7.2). There's a bit of a crossover with the large trapezius muscle that stretches down from the neck, crosses the shoulder blades, and finishes off in the upper back. Therefore, if you're having pain in between your shoulder blades then take a look at Chapter 5 on the neck as well, as that's where the trapezius muscle is covered.

I see a lot of clients with upper back problems because, as well as being very common, they're also difficult to treat by yourself. The space between our shoulder blades is one of the most difficult to reach, so you will probably have to go to a therapist for treatment or ask a friend or family member to massage the area for you.

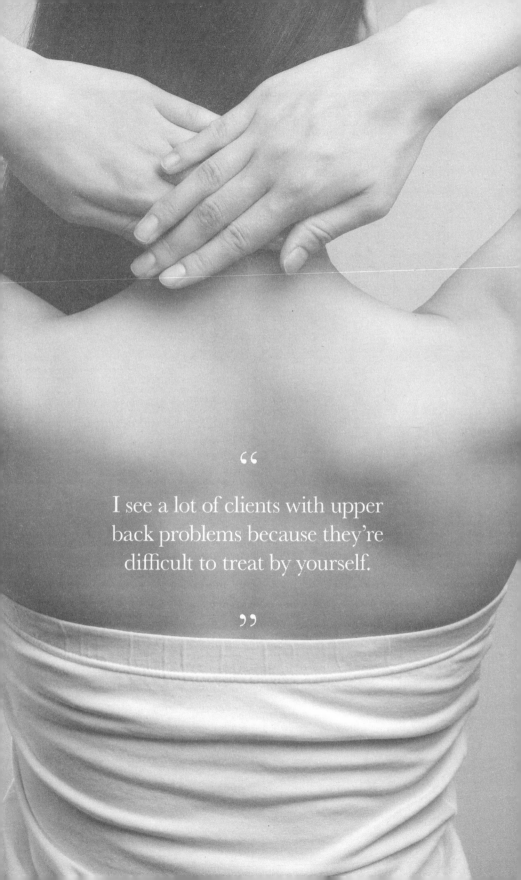

" I see a lot of clients with upper back problems because they're difficult to treat by yourself. "

FIG. 7.1
SECTIONS OF THE SPINE

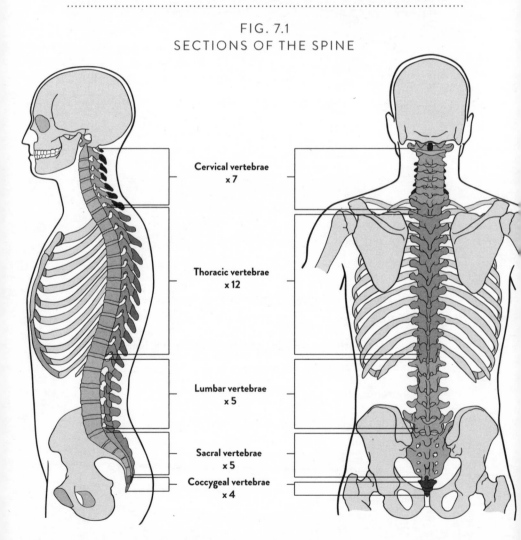

Cervical vertebrae
x 7

Thoracic vertebrae
x 12

Lumbar vertebrae
x 5

Sacral vertebrae
x 5

Coccygeal vertebrae
x 4

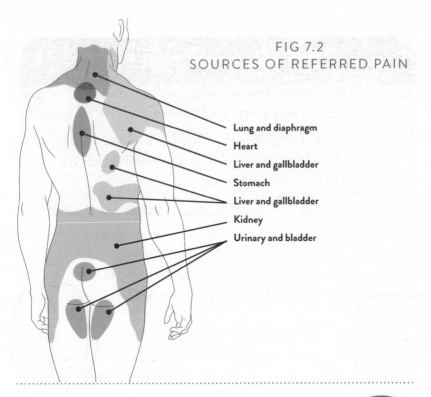

FIG 7.2
SOURCES OF REFERRED PAIN

Lung and diaphragm

Heart

Liver and gallbladder

Stomach

Liver and gallbladder

Kidney

Urinary and bladder

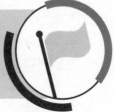

We should be aware of several warning flags when it comes to the upper back so always seek urgent medical attention if you experience any of the following:

- Chest pain that includes tightness or pressure to the chest area

- Difficulty breathing, including shortness of breath, being unable to talk properly, or gasping

- An extreme, sharp pain in the middle of the back

- Coughing that lasts for weeks and has an associated mid-back pain

- Pain in your upper back and a history of cancer

- An accident or trauma.

MOST COMMON UPPER BACK CONDITIONS: MUSCLE STRAIN

Clients usually come to me with a nagging pain in the upper back that they can't reach. There are lots of muscles in the upper back, but the good news is that they rarely tear. When I do see a tear in this area, it's almost always people who are serious about weightlifting. If that's not you, then you can usually rule out a tear.

The main muscle that is strained is the trapezius that stretches down from the neck, but it can often be some of the other superficial muscles around the shoulder blades, or even the deeper ones (see Figure 7.3).

Joints locking in the upper back are not as common as they are in the lower back and neck, so if you experience a dull ache in this area, it's more likely to be a muscle strain or rib problem, rather than a spinal issue.

Upper-back strain is usually the result of poor posture, lack of strength in the muscles (deconditioning), or repetitive overuse of the muscles. Posture problems usually occur because of slouching when working at a desk or driving.

A muscle strain in the upper back is really common and because of the low-level ache – often rated as a two or three on the pain scale – most people just ignore it and work through the pain. But muscle

PATIENT FILES: MUSCLE STRAIN

Joshua had strained his deep rhomboid muscles when I first met him. He was in his early thirties, looked fit and healthy, but hadn't done any exercise for ten years when he then decided to join a gym. His personal trainer had overestimated his strength and, not wanting to admit he wasn't as strong as he looked, Joshua lifted some weights and suffered a severe strain that was very painful. Luckily, the muscle hadn't torn, so his recovery was a lot quicker than if it had been. The key to his recovery was rest and I helped this with dry needling and alternating between massage and ice.

strains shouldn't be ignored because they can easily lead to joint and rib problems. The damage can also stray out of the upper back and start putting pressure on your shoulders, neck, and lower back. If this starts happening then the repercussions can be huge. I tore the quad muscle in my leg because I ignored a muscle strain in my lower back.

FIG. 7.3
SUPERFICIAL AND DEEP MUSCLES
IN THE UPPER BACK

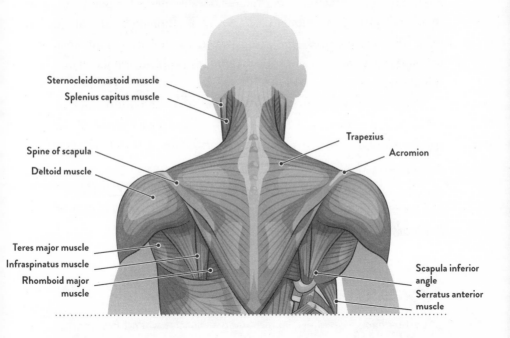

Sternocleidomastoid muscle
Splenius capitus muscle
Spine of scapula
Deltoid muscle
Teres major muscle
Infraspinatus muscle
Rhomboid major muscle
Trapezius
Acromion
Scapula inferior angle
Serratus anterior muscle

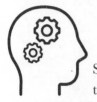

Start with your pain scale and **STOP**, and then consider the following:

- **S**ite: Usually between the shoulder blades and the mid-section of the spine.

- **T**ype: Spasm, tightness, dull ache, or stiffness.

- **Onset:** A gradual ache or stiffness that will normally come on over time. It can either be deep or superficial depending on which muscle it is (see Figure 7.3). It can sometimes be sudden if you have lifted something awkwardly, or reached for something in an unusual way.

- **Provoked:** It can be provoked by certain movements or staying in the posture that you suspect might have caused the strain, such as sitting at a desk, standing, or carrying a heavy bag to work.

> A referred pain from an organ can sometimes feel like an upper-back strain. The best way to tell the difference is to think about what provokes it. Does it get worse after you have eaten? Take a look at the 'Other Common Conditions' section in Chapter 10, 'The Abdomen', if you suspect this is a possibility.

HEAVY BAGS

If you carry a heavy bag regularly, ask someone to take a photo of you carrying it. You might be surprised at how much it pulls your posture to one side. Think about an alternative – once the root cause is removed, the strain normally goes away.

SELF-HELP

- Massage guns and foam rollers work really well on the upper back to achieve a deep pressure, and you can use these at home. When using a massage gun, be careful not to place it directly on the spine.

- A self-massage technique that you can do by yourself is to place a tennis ball on the floor and lie down on it with your upper back on top of the ball. Use your back to manoeuvre the ball over your muscles for a deep massage.

- You can go to an osteopath, physiotherapist, chiropractor or massage therapist for treatment. The therapist will use massage and mobilization to relieve the strain. They will need to work on the neck and shoulder, as well as the upper back. You might also need strengthening exercises if the strain is because of deconditioning (lack of strength in the muscles).

- With a muscle strain I would go through each rib and stretch it out, using the client's arm as a lever. Often the muscles between the ribs get very tight and this eases any tension there.

- In my experience, cupping is also very good for the upper back.

RIBS

Both women and men have twelve pairs of ribs. Some people are born with an extra rib above their collarbone that is called a *cervical rib*. It's usually harmless, but can be painful if it irritates a nerve. In my experience the ribs are the hardest area of the body to treat. Rib pain is usually because of one of the following three conditions:

- A rib is out of sync;

- The muscles in between the ribs are in spasm;

- A rib is fractured.

A rib fracture will usually only happen because of trauma such as a fall or car accident. It takes a lot of a force to break a rib, so there will be an unusual event preceding it.

An out-of-sync rib usually happens over time due to poor posture or repetitive movements. The rib won't be as supple as it should be, and this will put added pressure on the other ribs. They'll try to compensate for one rib's lack of mobility and eventually a rib will shift out of sync. Normally, if you have an issue with your ribs, your chest will also be tight, and you will need to work on opening it up.

Both conditions can be incredibly painful, but the pain from a fracture tends to be constant, whereas clients with an out-of-sync rib have told me that it's usually a twisting movement or bending forwards that brings on the pain.

PATIENT FILES: RIBS

Jenny came to see me after spending months going to a massage therapist to try and get rid of the knots across the top of her back. She'd been having lots of deep-tissue massages and had accepted that these were going to be more painful than a lighter massage. She'd therefore had hours of massage, with elbows digging into her muscles.

I examined her back and she was relieved to hear that she didn't actually have lots of knots in her back – the bumps were, in fact, her ribs. I worked at stretching out the front of her ribs and left her back alone (it had already had enough treatment). The pain across her back lessened. It was the tightness in her ribs that had caused the generalized pain across her back.

In between each rib there is a thick band of muscles called the intercostal muscles (Figure 7.4), which make up your chest wall. These muscles help your ribcage expand and contract when you breathe. When these muscles become tight, they can make breathing painful and even lead to problems with your ribs, so they should be loosened up. I've had several clients come to me after going for a Thai massage. The massage therapist walked on the client's back to try and loosen up these muscles and instead, a rib shifted out of sync. If you're ever in doubt: the back is not really designed to be walked on and there should be a strong rationale behind performing this treatment.

Even your breathing can put strain on the ribs and intercostal muscles if you are breathing from your chest rather than your diaphragm. Often when I see clients, they have to work on relearning how to breathe through the lower belly, which should rise when you inhale rather than the chest. There's more about this in Chapter 18.

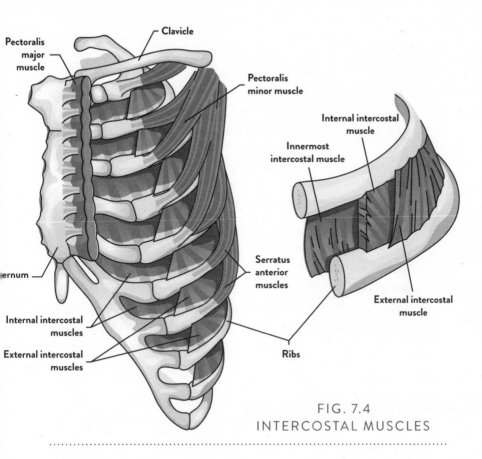

Pectoralis major muscle

Clavicle

Pectoralis minor muscle

Internal intercostal muscle

Innermost intercostal muscle

Sternum

Serratus anterior muscles

Internal intercostal muscles

External intercostal muscles

External intercostal muscle

Ribs

FIG. 7.4
INTERCOSTAL MUSCLES

Start with your pain scale and **STOP**, and then consider the following:

- **S**ite: Localized to the site of the rib. Sometimes rib pain can be a referred pain to the front and side of the chest.

- **T**ype: Can be a very sharp, acute pain if the injury is fresh, or it can be a dull, background ache that gets worse with movement. A fractured rib will usually mean constant pain.

- **O**nset: It can be gradual or sudden. A fractured rib will normally only happen with trauma.

- **P**rovoked: Twisting actions, breathing, or bending.

SELF-HELP

- Stretching out the ribs helps considerably with the intercostal muscles, and this can be done by a skilled therapist. Alternatively, at home, you can practise the exercise to open up your chest that is at the end of this chapter.

PROFESSIONAL HELP

- Ribs are very difficult to treat so you should see either an osteopath or chiropractor, who is highly skilled and experienced in treating ribs.

- If the rib is out of sync, then it will normally need to be clicked back into the correct position. Please don't try this at home as even for a therapist with training in anatomy this is very difficult to do – the movement has to be very precise or it can do more damage.

- The therapist should locate the rib in question and work on the muscles around it. If the rib is out of sync it will need to be clicked back. This only needs to be done on the rib in question and the therapist shouldn't click the rest of the ribs as well.

- If the pain from an intercostal muscle is very acute it might be that the client can't stand to have the area touched. In these cases, I spend time loosing up the neck, diaphragm, and shoulders before moving on to the ribs. Dry needling also really helps with rib pain.

If breathing brings on pain, then it's likely you've got a rib out of sync, or a fractured rib.

The pain from rib problems is usually to one side and sometimes follows the angle of the rib.

OTHER COMMON UPPER-BACK CONDITIONS

- *Damage to a disc*, such as a disc bulge or herniated disc, is less common in the thoracic spine than the neck or lower back, but it happens. A damaged disc in this area doesn't usually cause pain or other symptoms, so often goes undiagnosed.

- *Compression fractures* in the spine are caused when a vertebra becomes weak and cannot support the weight of the body above it. Small fractures will develop, which can cause the spine to shrink and lead to pain from a resulting change to posture.

- Both *rheumatoid arthritis and osteoarthritis* can happen in the thoracic spine. See Chapter 3 for more information.

- *Scoliosis* is a condition where the spine curves and twists to the side. It can sometimes make the spine curve in an 'S' shape when seen from the back, rather than the side. It can be mild or, in extreme cases, require surgery. Signs of it are differing shoulder heights, clothes not hanging correctly, and the person leaning to the side.

STRETCHES AND EXERCISES FOR UPPER BACK

The upper back is difficult to get to so these have all been selected as things you can do by yourself. As with all the exercises in the book, if they are painful or make your injury worse then please stop them immediately.

FIG. 7.5.
CHILD'S POSE

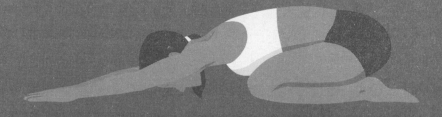

1

You can try some self-massage
with a foam roller. These are
cheap to buy compared to a
massage gun and worth investing
in. Place the foam roller on the
ground so it is positioned across
the width of your back. Lie down
with the top half of your back on
the foam roller. Support your neck
with your hands behind the back
of your head. Bend your knees so
your body is lifted off the ground
and use your bent legs to gently
roll your back over the foam roller.
Your back might click when you
do this, but it's nothing to be
worried about.

2

The *Child's Pose* in yoga (see
Figure 7.5) is very good at
releasing tension from the spine
and stretching your latissimus
dorsi muscles, which are the
large muscles that run above
and below your waist. From a
kneeling position, sit back on your
feet and lower your body so your
head is close to the floor in front
of your knees. Stretch out your
arms all the way in front of your
head, keep your neck in a relaxed
position and your head facing the
floor. Hold the position for around
twenty seconds.

FIG. 7.6
THREAD THE NEEDLE

FIG. 7.7
'W' POSITION

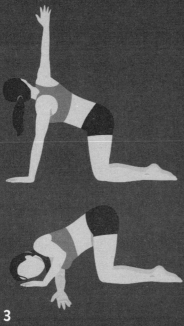

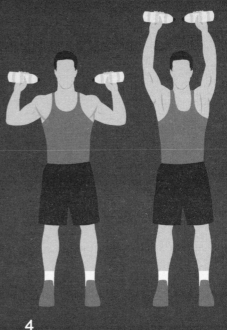

3

Thread the Needle (see Figure 7.6) is another yoga pose that is great for stretching the latissimus dorsi muscles and the muscles in the upper back. It's also really good for increasing mobility in the thoracic spine. Start on your hands and knees, with your arms directly below your shoulders. Take your left arm and pass it through the gap between your shoulder and legs, while rotating your chest. Keep the palm of your left arm face-up and lower your left shoulder towards the floor. Stretch your right arm out in front of you and let your head rest on the floor looking towards the ceiling. Hold this position for twenty seconds before switching to the other side.

4

Opening up your chest helps combat those rounded shoulders. This exercise doesn't require any gym equipment and can therefore be done in an office. While standing, hold your arms out and above your head as if in a ten-to-two position on a clock. Hold this for five seconds. Lower your arms to the 'W' position in Figure 7.7 and squeeze your shoulder blades together for two seconds. Switch between the two movements two or three times.

CHAPTER 8

Elbow

The elbow joint is more complicated than most of us realize because it connects the single bone in our upper arm with the two bones in our forearms (see Figure 8.1). It's therefore made up of three joints that allow us to pull our forearm backwards and forwards, as well as rotate it. The elbow is known as a hinge joint, similar to the ones in your knee and ankle. Most of us recognize that the elbow joint allows us to do a bicep curl, but it's often overlooked that it also allows us to turn a door handle.

MYTH BUSTERS

The funny bone isn't a bone or even part of one. That sharp pain you feel when you whack your elbow is from knocking the ulnar nerve that runs through a ridge of your humerus bone – which gives the funny bone its name.

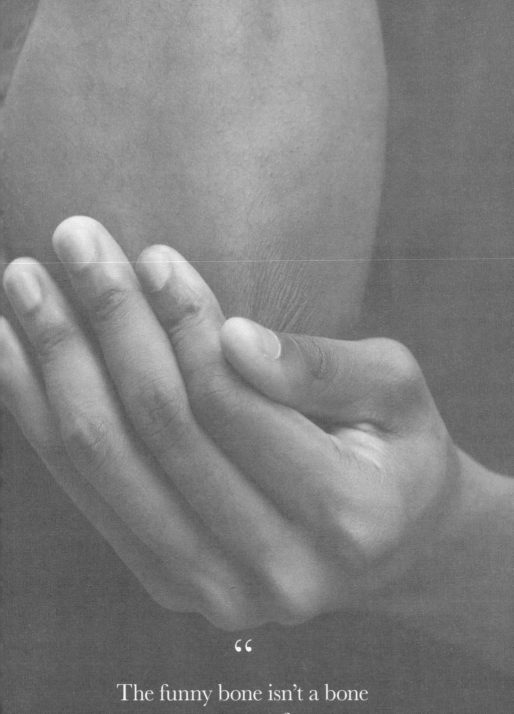

"

The funny bone isn't a bone
or even part of one.

"

FIG. 8.1
ANATOMY OF ELBOW

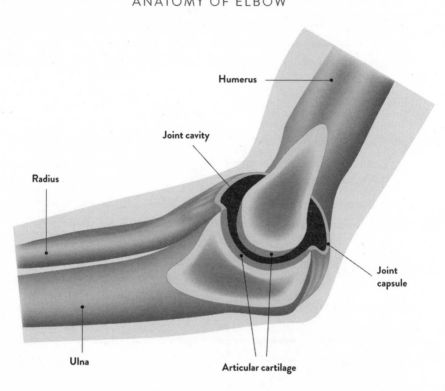

Humerus

Joint cavity

Radius

Joint capsule

Ulna

Articular cartilage

SYMPTOMS

CHECK

ARE YOUR ELBOWS HEALTHY?

With a healthy elbow you should
be able to do the following:

1
Fully straighten your
arm

2
Bend your elbow so
you can touch the
tip of your shoulder
with your hand

3
Twist your forearm
with the palm facing
up to the palm
facing down, and
vice versa

Our forearm muscles are surprisingly strong and are constantly used in activities involving our elbows, wrist, or hands. Irritation of the tendons that link the forearm muscles to the elbow joints is the most common problem in the elbow, which are known as tennis elbow and golfer's elbow. Despite their names, I don't have a succession of golfers and tennis players coming through my doors with these problems. Instead, it's usually people who have manual jobs or work with their hands such as tilers, musicians, and secretaries.

There are a couple of (hopefully) one-off injuries to the elbow that I should mention quickly, which are a dislocated elbow and a fractured elbow. With both of these you should know that they are a possibility if you've have had a fall or been in a car accident. A fractured elbow will be swollen, you'll have difficulty moving it, and there may also be a lump underneath the skin. You might still be able to move the elbow with a fracture, depending on where it is, so it's best to have an X-ray immediately to check this. If the joint is dislocated, it will feel loose and floppy. Both are very painful and require immediate medical treatment, like the other warning flags below.

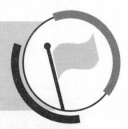

There are several warning flags when it comes to the elbow so always seek urgent medical attention if you experience any of the following:

- The joint is red, hot or swollen, and movement has reduced

- Both elbows are painful

- You have been involved in an accident or suffered trauma

- There is a mass or lump that is growing in size

MOST COMMON ELBOW CONDITIONS : TENNIS ELBOW AND GOLFER'S ELBOW

Both tennis elbow and golfer's elbow happen when the muscles in the forearms are overworked, which causes inflammation in the tendons that attach to the elbow joint (see Figures 8.2a and b). These conditions often occur when people do the same motion throughout the day. The key difference between the two is that pain from tennis elbow is on the outside of the elbow joint, whereas golfer's elbow is on the inside.

Tennis elbow occurs when you regularly stretch the wrist backwards or spread your fingers. Golfer's elbow comes from bending the wrist forwards or gripping things. They are pretty much opposite motions from each other. From my experience, tennis elbow is more common than golfer's elbow.

PATIENT FILES: TENNIS ELBOW

Matt worked part-time as a musician, playing the bass guitar. If he wasn't performing at a gig in the evening, he practised for three hours every night. He came to me because he had tennis elbow and was avoiding playing his guitar as it hurt too much. I examined him and it was clear that his forearm muscles were strained, but that this was the root cause of the problem. Before I started treating the elbow with my hands, I gave him some dry needling around the forearm muscles and massaged his wrists as they were tired from overuse. Next was a massage of the upper arm and shoulder. By now the elbow was less tender and I was able to do some gentle mobilization on it. He was then able to take a couple of weeks off from playing the guitar. Matt now treats his guitar playing as if he is an athlete and warms up his arms and wrists beforehand. The problem hasn't returned.

The people who come to see me with either of these conditions use their hands a lot – for example, manual workers, decorators, plasterers, typists, chefs, butchers, and so on – and usually don't play golf or tennis. They are normally over the age of 30, as the condition can take a while to develop, and because of the initial low-level pain, people tend not to do anything about it until it becomes so painful that it's tender to touch. In my experience, I see more men with these conditions than women.

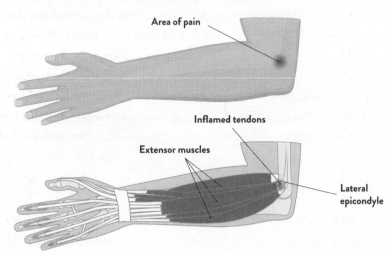

FIG. 8.2A
TENNIS ELBOW (LATERAL EPICONDYLITIS)

Area of pain

Inflamed tendons

Extensor muscles

Lateral epicondyle

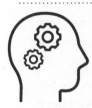

TENNIS ELBOW

For tennis elbow, start with your pain scale and **STOP**, and then consider the following:

- **S**ite: Pain will be on the outside of the elbow. If it worsens, it might travel down the forearm.

- **T**ype: An aching pain. There will usually be stiffness and swelling and some clients have told me it feels like a burning pain (which is normally used to describe nerve pain, but this is one of those rare times that tissue pain feels like nerve pain). There may also be a weakness in the grip.

- **O**nset: It will be a gradual onset, but there might be sudden pain if there is a new micro-tear in the tendon.

- **P**rovoked by: Moving the wrist backwards or gripping things. Twisting the forearm to turn a handle or open a jar.

FIG. 8.2B

GOLFER'S ELBOW (MEDIAL EPICONDYLITIS)

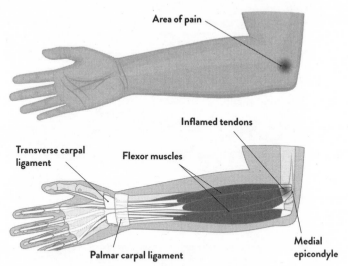

Area of pain

Inflamed tendons

Transverse carpal ligament

Flexor muscles

Medial epicondyle

Palmar carpal ligament

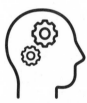

GOLFER'S ELBOW

For golfer's elbow, start with your pain scale and **STOP**, and then consider the following:

- **S**ite: Pain will be on the inside of the elbow. If it gets worse it might travel down the forearm. Sometimes there can be a tingling sensation from the elbow to the hand.

- **T**ype: An aching pain, accompanied by stiffness, swelling, or weakness in the grip. Some clients have told me that it can feel like a burning pain at times.

- **O**nset: It will be a gradual onset, but there might be a sudden pain if there is a new micro-tear in the tendon.

- **P**rovoked by: Moving the wrist forwards or gripping things. Twisting the forearm inwards.

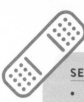

- Patients are often advised that they should strengthen their forearm muscles when they have either golfer's elbow or tennis elbow, but I believe that the forearms are already very strong and just need time to recover. Rest is important for these types of injuries, if you can take it.

- If you're treating this at home, I would try self-massage with some oil. It's best to work on the area of the forearm that is a couple of centimetres away from the site of the pain and do small circular massages, before massaging down the length of the forearm.

PROFESSIONAL HELP

- Either of these conditions will heal by themselves if you stop doing the repetitive movement that caused them. For most people this isn't an option, as it is required by their jobs, so treatment from a therapist usually helps speed up the recovery.

- If there is a limitation of movement, and it's not too painful to touch, I would massage and mobilize the area around the joint, but also work on the entire arm, including the wrist, hand, forearm, and shoulder. It's never as simple as just one site being tight; it might be that the biceps, triceps, or forearm muscles are tight as well.

- If the elbow is too painful to touch, then cold laser therapy can be a useful treatment as long as it doesn't aggravate the pain.

- Dry needling away from the site can also be useful. I would usually do this around the forearms as they have been overused and are the actual cause of the problem. For tennis elbow this is around the extensors on the outside of the forearm, and for golfer's elbow it is the flexors, which are on the inside of the forearm. I would also use electroacupuncture on the site of the tendon.

- It might be that the elbow joint needs to be clicked back into place. If this is necessary, then the therapist should try mobilization first to return it to the right place before resorting to clicking.

- If the problem doesn't resolve, you might decide to get a steroid injection, which would be arranged by your doctor.

ELBOW SPRAIN AND TEAR

Sprains can also happen through overuse of the arms from repetitive movements. Both tears and sprains can be extremely painful and often mean you can't straighten your arm properly. A tear can either be partial or full. The good news is that most people will make a full recovery from a simple elbow sprain within four weeks.

> ### PATIENT FILES: SPRAIN
>
> From Chapter 3 we know that sprains affect ligaments rather than muscles and tendons. Sprains and tears to the elbow ligaments normally happen when the arm is bent or twisted quickly, so they usually involve a fall or sporting injury, but they can also happen when you carry too much. This was what happened to my client, Dan, when he lifted some weights at the gym that were too heavy for him. He felt a really sharp pain in his elbow and noticed afterwards that it was swelling up and he couldn't straighten it fully.

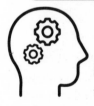

Start with your pain scale and **STOP**, and then consider the following:

- **S**ite: Where the ligament is that has been damaged.

- **T**ype: If a ligament is sprained it will be tender to touch, as well as swollen, and there will be a severe ache. If it is torn, it will usually swell up very quickly and the skin will be red. Clients have described a 'pinging' sensation when their ligament tears, accompanied by a sharp pain. There may also be a popping sound when moving an elbow with a ligament tear and it will usually also feel weak.

- **O**nset: It will be sudden if it's a tear. For a sprain it can be gradual or sudden, depending on whether it occurred because of trauma or overuse.

- **P**rovoked: It will be more painful when bending or straightening the elbow.

SELF-HELP

When the injury is inflamed try **R**est, **I**ce, **C**ompression, and **E**levation (see page 70).

PROFESSIONAL HELP

- You can see an osteopath, chiropractor or physiotherapist for treatment.

- Dry needling around the site of the ligament works really well for a sprain or tear.

- For both a sprain or a tear you might need to wear a sling, or even have a brace if the damage is very bad.

- If the ligament is ruptured (a complete tear), then you will probably need surgery. It's important that after surgery you follow the physiotherapy recommendations that the hospital provides.

OTHER COMMON ELBOW CONDITIONS

- *Olecranon bursitis* is an inflammation of the bursa on the back of the elbow joint. It will normally be quite red and puffy. There may also be tenderness and pain when leaning on the elbow.

- *Osteoarthritis* is quite common in the elbow joint. The joint will often make a creaking noise and there may be swelling when it has been present for a while. There might also be stiffness in the joint for a short time in the morning. It will normally only be in one elbow.

- *Rheumatoid Arthritis* will normally occur in both elbows. There will be stiffness and restricted movement. Other joints might be affected as well.

- *Bicep tendon strain.* The bicep is the large muscle at the front of the upper arm. It is quite common for the tendon at the bottom of the bicep, which attaches over the front of the elbow joint, to become strained or even tear.

STRETCHES AND EXERCISES FOR THE ELBOW

If you've read any of the other chapters on specific areas of the body, you will have noticed that at the end of each chapter, I have listed lots of exercises and stretches to help strengthen that area of the body. With the injuries to the elbow that I've mentioned above, I actually believe that they will benefit from rest, rather than exercise. Try and rest those tired arms if you can. Saying that, some gentle movements of the joint may help if you support it at the same time. It's therefore important to do the following while pressing on the muscle or joint in question with your other hand, as shown in Figure. 8.3. As with all the exercises in the book, if they are painful or make your injury worse then please stop them immediately:

FIG. 8.3
EXERCISE FOR THE ELBOW

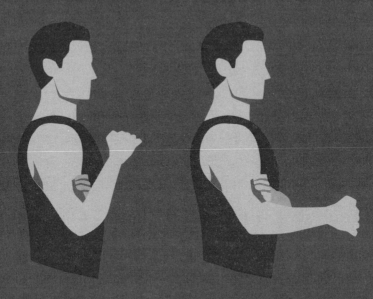

1

Curl your arm up and press down with your other hand on the biceps and triceps to support them. Gently extend your forearm and then bring it back to your shoulder again if you can. Repeat this ten times on both sides.

2

Do the same action as above but this time pressing down on one side of the elbow joint or both sides using the thumb on one side and your finger pads on the other.

CHAPTER 9

Wrist
and hand

Before we get into their anatomy, I want to take a moment to appreciate how dexterous our hands are because of their opposable thumbs, long fingers, and the development of a pincer grip. They allow us to grasp and handle objects in such a finely tuned way that we were eventually able to make complex tools. There are over twenty-seven bones in each of your hands, including your wrists, and 206 bones in the human body, so both of your hands account for around 26 per cent of your bones. So, before we start on the hands, just think for a moment of how much they do for us and where we would be without them.

After a few years of using my hands constantly throughout the day, kneading client's muscles and mobilizing their joints, they had begun to ache at about a two on the pain scale. I therefore devised a massage routine for my hands, wrists, and forearms that I now do every day, usually when I'm waiting for the kettle to boil or my toast to pop out of the toaster. I also dry needle the muscles in my forearms twice a month, to help prevent any injuries from occurring. Just kneading the ropey parts of your forearm muscles will help. These routines have enabled me to carry on working pain-free for another ten years, and there will be more about this in the exercises section at the end of the chapter.

"
Take a moment to appreciate
how dexterous our hands are.
"

The hand's large range of movement and ability to use fine motor skills comes from all the bones, muscles, and tendons. As you'll see from the diagram of the hands in Figure 9.1, there are many fine bones that help control the movements of your fingers and these make it a unique part of the body.

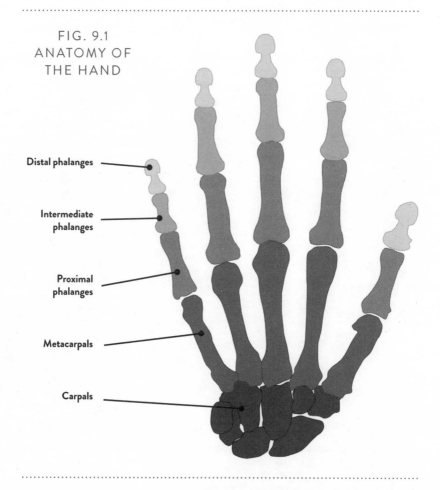

FIG. 9.1
ANATOMY OF
THE HAND

Distal phalanges

Intermediate phalanges

Proximal phalanges

Metacarpals

Carpals

Our hands can also clearly show us if there is something wrong with one of the nerves that travel into them. We can even identify which nerve it is just from the shape our hand makes (see Figure 9.2). If your hand has started to curl, then you should check to see if the median, ulnar, or radial nerves have been affected.

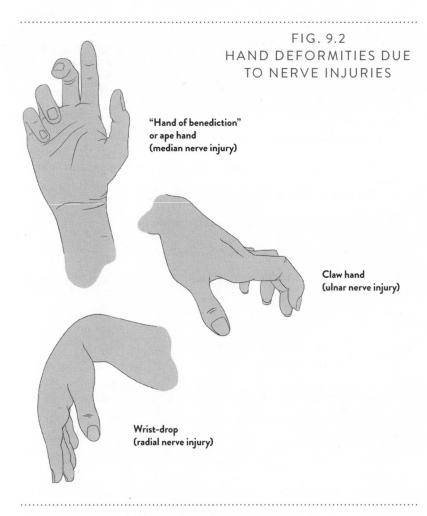

FIG. 9.2
HAND DEFORMITIES DUE
TO NERVE INJURIES

"Hand of benediction"
or ape hand
(median nerve injury)

Claw hand
(ulnar nerve injury)

Wrist-drop
(radial nerve injury)

The wrists are the bridge between the forearms and hands and contain eight bones. I usually treat the wrist and hands as one, as they are so interlinked, and strain on one will often cause problems in the other.

The people I normally see with problems with their hands are usually over the age of 40, but they can obviously appear at any age depending on what the condition is.

People with wrist conditions span all ages, as they are usually due to trauma or carpal tunnel syndrome, which can begin as early as your twenties.

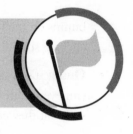

There are several warning flags when it comes to the wrists and hands so always seek urgent medical attention if you experience any of the following:

- A quickly expanding, painful lump on the hand

- Weakness and limited movement in both hands or wrists

- The wrist is very red, puffy, or swollen

- Inability to bend or straighten the wrist at all

- An infection in the wrist and inability to move it

- A fall or trauma to the wrist or hand (such as when I slammed the boot of a car on my hand!)

MOST COMMON HAND AND WRIST CONDITIONS: ARTHRITIS

In my experience, the hands are one of the most common places to have arthritis. Rheumatoid arthritis is normally found in the knuckles and in both hands, whereas osteoarthritis is usually in one hand and affects the end joints of the fingers. There is more about arthritis in Chapter 3.

OSTEOARTHRITIS

For osteoarthritis, start with your pain scale and **STOP**, and then consider the following:

- **S**ite: Usually in the base of the thumb where it is linked to the wrist, or it can be in the middle or end joints of the fingers. It can be in one or both hands, but tends to just be in one (see Figure 9.3).

- **T**ype: Often described as sore or achy, but can be painless as well. If there is pain, it can range from mild to severe. There will normally be stiffness in the joints that can start to form lumps or bumps on the fingers. When moved, there can be a creaking or clicking sound.

- **O**nset: It's progressive and over time it usually gets worse. There can eventually be a constant sharp pain and the fingers will be so stiff that they cannot fully bend.

- **P**rovoked: The stiffness usually worsens from inactivity and cold weather. The pain is often briefly worse in the mornings, usually improves when you start to move, and then can get worse again at the end of the day. People with osteoarthritis will usually have difficulty with everyday tasks such as using a phone, buttoning a shirt, gripping objects, opening a jar, or turning a key.

FIG. 9.3
OSTEOARTHRITIS IN HANDS

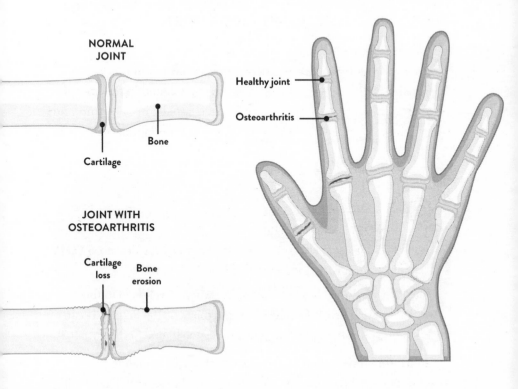

NORMAL
JOINT

Healthy joint

Osteoarthritis

Bone

Cartilage

JOINT WITH
OSTEOARTHRITIS

Cartilage
loss

Bone
erosion

Osteoarthritis is more common in women than men. When it affects the hands, it often runs in families. If your mother or grandmother has lumps on their hands, then it's more likely you will also have them when you get older.

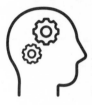

RHEUMATOID ARTHRITIS

For rheumatoid arthritis, start with your pain scale and **STOP**, and then consider the following:

- **S**ite: Commonly starts with pain in the hand, wrists, and toes, and then spreads to the other joints. The pain occurs simultaneously on both hands/wrists and other joints.

- **T**ype: The joints look red, hot, and swollen. There may also be a discolouration of the joints.

- **O**nset: It normally begins without you realizing, but even when it is asymptomatic, damage will be happening to your joints. It usually starts when people are aged between 20 and 55.

- **P**rovoked: The pain can be worse in the mornings, lasting for over thirty minutes and possibly even hours.

Women are two to three times more likely to suffer from rheumatoid arthritis than men.

With rheumatoid arthritis there are associated symptoms of fatigue, a general feeling of discomfort, and depression.

If rheumatoid arthritis in the hands becomes advanced, then there can be visible changes to the shape of the hand (see Figure 9.4.).

FIG. 9.4

CHANGES TO SHAPE OF HAND FROM RHEUMATOID ARTHRITIS

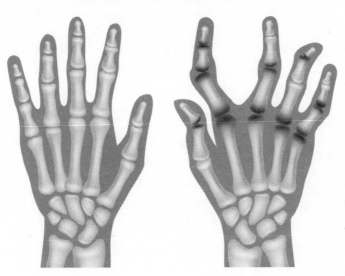

NORMAL   RHUMATOID ARTHRITIS

SELF-HELP

- Massage to the tiny muscles in the fingers and hand can be beneficial, as well as general circling motions of the palms and wrists.

- A lot of the massage techniques can be done at home, but you will probably need a friend or relative to help with this if your arthritis is advanced.

PROFESSIONAL HELP

- Rheumatoid arthritis is normally treated with immuno-suppressant medication, or occasionally a steroid injection for short-term treatment, by a doctor. For both osteoarthritis and rheumatoid arthritis an osteopath, physiotherapist, or chiropractor can help with mobilizing the joints. It's good to try and keep the hands moving in these cases as when you rest them, they become stiffer.

FIG. 9.5

CARPAL TUNNEL SYNDROME VS. ARTHRITIS

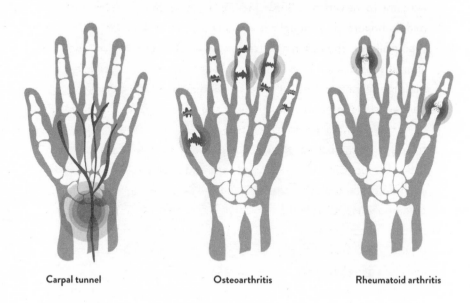

Carpal tunnel   Osteoarthritis   Rheumatoid arthritis

CARPAL TUNNEL SYNDROME

Most people have heard of carpal tunnel syndrome, but what they probably don't know is that the carpal tunnel is actually an area of the wrist. It's a passageway for tendons, nerves, and blood vessels to travel through to the hand. Carpal tunnel syndrome is when this tunnel becomes swollen and presses on the median nerve passing through it. Several nerves serve very specific areas of your hands, so if you are experiencing altered sensations in your hands then check Figure 9.6 to see which nerve it might be that is damaged.

I often see clients with carpal tunnel syndrome who type, play musical instruments, or use tools a lot, particularly vibrating ones. They tend to mostly be women over the age of 50, pregnant women, or people with diabetes.

PATIENT FILES: CARPAL TUNNEL SYNDROME

Ali came to me with numbness and tingling in her thumb, index, and middle fingers. She thought it was a repetitive strain injury from typing all day. She was in her late thirties and had experienced the altered sensations for several years. I examined her and used the massage technique I use for the carpal tunnel, as well as treating her hands and forearms. I asked her if she also had pain in the back of her neck and she confirmed that she did. The median nerve travels from the base of the neck and where it exited her spine it had got trapped in a strained muscle and stiffened joint. This was in addition to the problems she had with the carpal tunnel – the two commonly happen together. I treated her neck by opening up the space where the median nerve exits the spine. She couldn't stop typing, as she had to do this for her job, but she started stretching and massaging her hands before work and her symptoms improved.

FIG. 9.6
THE THREE NERVES THAT
SUPPLY THE HANDS

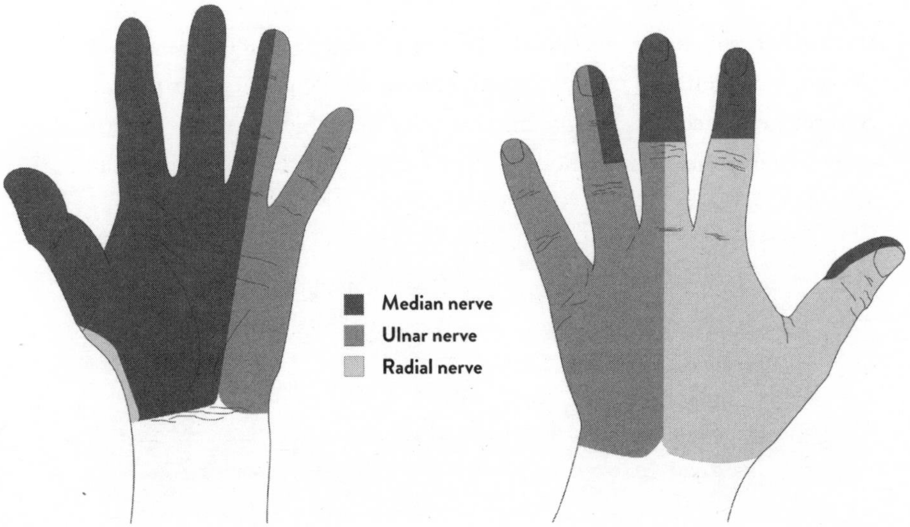

Median nerve
Ulnar nerve
Radial nerve

A way of testing for carpal tunnel syndrome is to shake your hands if there is a numb or tingling sensation. This will make these sensations briefly go away as it increases the blood flow and reduces the internal swelling.

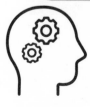

Start with your pain scale and **STOP**, and then consider the following:

- **S**ite: Symptoms can typically be in the hand, some fingers (the first three: thumb, index finger, and middle finger), the wrist, or forearm.

- **T**ype: If there is pain, then it will be an aching pain. There will also be intermittent tingling, numbness, or weakness.

- **O**nset: It will be a gradual onset.

- **P**rovoked: Usually provoked by doing the repetitive action that has caused the problem and is often worse at night. In more severe cases it will be difficult to grip objects and you might find that you are dropping things.

SELF-HELP

A really useful technique I use for stretching the carpal tunnel wall is to take the client's hand with their palm facing upwards in both of my hands. I place my thumbs at the base of the client's hand and firmly pull both my thumbs in opposite directions across the palm to the edge of the hand (see Figure 9.7). This is one of the best techniques for carpal tunnel syndrome and can be transformative when done regularly. I'll also massage around the forearm muscles as well – if these are loosened, it takes pressure off the tendons in the hands. You can ask a friend or family member to do this for you.

FIG. 9.7
MASSAGE FOR CARPAL TUNNEL SYNDROME

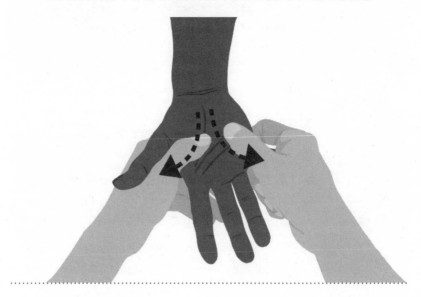

PROFESSIONAL HELP

- You can see an osteopath, physiotherapist or chiropractor for treatment. You might be offered a wrist splint from your doctor.

- When I treat carpal tunnel syndrome, I always trace the median nerve up through the arm and shoulder and to the neck, and work on the tight muscles in these regions. The numbness in the hands or tingling might actually be from the compression of the median nerve body instead of in the carpal tunnel, or it might be a dual compression – one in the carpal tunnel and also further up, usually in the shoulder or neck.

- It might be that you need a carpal bone clicked back into place but, as with all clicking, this should only be done if necessary, and the therapist should try mobilization first.

- People are often offered surgery with carpal tunnel syndrome, but I've seen many people recover with just the massage technique above and not need surgery in the end. I would personally leave surgery until all other treatment avenues have been exhausted.

OTHER COMMON WRIST AND HAND CONDITIONS

- *Repetitive Strain Injury* (RSI) is a general term for a strain to muscles, tendons, and nerves that is caused by repeating the same movements. It's usually an achy type of pain from overuse. Treatment will depend on where the problem is, but it's not something to ignore as it will usually get worse.

- *Dupuytren's Contracture* is when the skin thickens on the palm of your hand just below your fingers, usually the ring and little fingers. It tends to be in older people and can even pull the fingers down towards the palm. Massage can help release the tightness in the palm. It's more common in men than women.

- *Ganglion cysts* are jelly-filled cysts that can form on the wrist joint. They are often harmless and just go away by themselves. If it does become painful you can go to your doctor to have it drained, or you may require surgery to remove it. You should never hit a ganglion with a book (or any other object) to try and break up the cyst.

STRETCHES AND EXERCISES FOR THE HANDS AND WRISTS

The hands really benefit from self-massage. In my experience it can help reduce pain and improve grip strength. Just kneading the palms of your hands in small circles can be beneficial and it's something you can do yourself when at work. There are also some stretches below you can do for the hands and wrists. As with all the exercises in the book, if they are painful or make your injury worse then please stop them immediately.

FIG. 9.8
PRAYER WRIST STRETCH

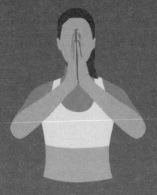 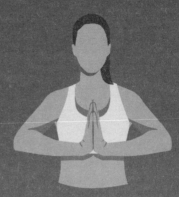

1

While standing, place your hands together in a prayer position in front of your face. Your arms should be touching each other from your finger to your elbows. With your palms still pressed together, lower your hands to your waist and slowly spread your elbows apart (see Figure 9.8). When you feel a stretch in your wrists hold the position for twenty seconds.

2

Hold one of your arms straight out at shoulder height with your hand facing the floor. Let your wrist drop your hand down. With the other hand gently pull your hand towards your body and hold the stretch for twenty seconds. Do this on the other arm as well.

3

To stretch your wrist the other way, hold your arm out again at shoulder height, but with your palm facing the sky. With the other hand gently press your fingers down towards the floor and then back towards your body. Hold for twenty seconds and then change to the other arm.

4

Lift your arms above your head. Interlace your fingers with your palms pressed together. Keeping your fingers interlaced, turn your palms up until they are facing the sky and hold the stretch. Repeat this a couple of times.

CHAPTER 10

Abdomen

Your abdomen and thorax house all your soft internal organs, which are collectively called the 'visceral organs'. It's where the essential workings of your body are conducted – for instance, your lungs breathe in air to enrich the blood with oxygen that is carried to your heart. The heart then pumps the blood around your body, while the digestive system breaks down your food so its nutrients can be absorbed into the blood stream. The beauty is in the continuity.

As an osteopath, I rarely treat clients with lung and heart conditions, but I do see a lot of clients who have problems with their digestion. It may also surprise you that osteopaths can help with digestive conditions, particularly constipation.

Most people think of digestion problems as diarrhoea or constipation but there are so many more symptoms that we need to be aware of (see Figure 10.1).

The digestive tract is not just your stomach and intestines. It runs all the way from your mouth down to the last sphincter muscle. It is made up of several organs that each play a role in digesting your food, extracting nutrients, and disposing of the waste product.

The digestive tract is considered to be our second brain as it has the same type of nerve cells as our brain. You wouldn't be able to work

"
It may surprise you that
osteopaths can help with
digestive conditions.
"

out the correct change at the supermarket with it, but there is direct communication between the brain and gut, and growing evidence that the gut may have an impact on our mood. For a long time, it's been known that anxiety and depression is linked to poor digestion. Originally, it was thought that anxiety and depression caused poor digestion, but now researchers are beginning to believe it is the other way around. If this is the case, it will revolutionize the way we think about what we eat.

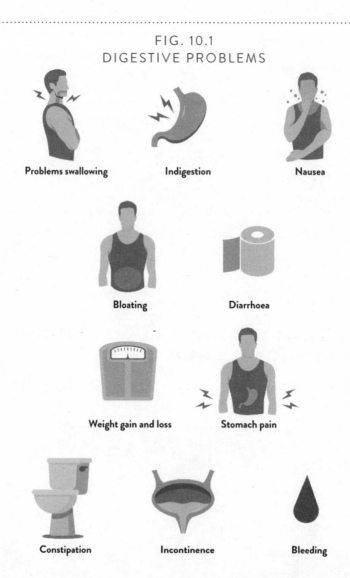

FIG. 10.1
DIGESTIVE PROBLEMS

Problems swallowing   Indigestion   Nausea

Bloating   Diarrhoea

Weight gain and loss   Stomach pain

Constipation   Incontinence   Bleeding

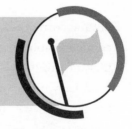

There are several warning flags when it comes to the abdomen so always seek urgent medical attention if you experience any of the following:

- Sudden abdominal pain

- Vomiting blood

- Change in bowel habits that lasts for more than three weeks

- Difficulty swallowing

- New discomfort or pain in the upper abdomen

- Persistent, unexplained vomiting

- Any swelling or enlargement of the abdomen

- Not passing wind

- Absolute constipation

- New lump or bump in the tummy

- Unexplained weight loss

- Change in stools, such as blood

- Your skin and the whites of your eyes have turned yellow

MOST COMMON ABDOMINAL CONDITIONS: IRRITABLE BOWEL SYNDROME (IBS)

Irritable Bowel Syndrome (IBS) is a general term for problems with the digestive system, particularly the small or large intestines. The symptoms vary with every patient, but it can include cramps, bloating, diarrhoea, and constipation. There isn't a specific test to confirm that you have IBS. Instead, it's a catch-all diagnosis a doctor will often make when other conditions that can be tested for have been ruled out. It's normally a life-long condition, and there is no cure, but it can be managed successfully with some lifestyle changes. Not a lot is known about IBS as it's such a wide-ranging condition, but it's thought that several things can trigger it such as food intolerances, stress, a gut infection, and antibiotics.

> ## PATIENT FILES: IBS
>
> Alisha had a nagging pain in her lower back that would come and go, and it was only from her patient history form that I realized that she also had IBS. Alisha hadn't mentioned it as she didn't know that osteopaths can help alleviate some of its symptoms. I used visceral massage techniques to reduce her bloating and decrease her sensitivity to touch in the area.

Most of the clients I see with IBS don't come to me because of it. Instead, they arrive at my doors with lower-back pain and won't have realized that the two are often connected. This is exactly what had happened to Alisha.

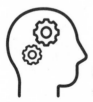

Start with your pain scale and **STOP**, and then consider the following:

- **S**ite: Most symptoms are in the stomach area, but there can also be pain in the lower back.

- **T**ype: There is usually pain associated with IBS and it has been described to me as cramping, aching, or sharp. Other common symptoms are bloating, swollen stomach, mucus in stools, gas, diarrhoea, constipation, lower-back pain, nausea, and fatigue.

- **O**nset: It's mainly intermittent and can last for a few days or months.

- **P**rovoked: It's often provoked after you've eaten certain foods. Usually, the pain gets better after passing a stool, but in some cases it can get worse.

IBS is different from constipation as there will be several of the symptoms listed above in **T**ype rather than just constipation.

SELF-HELP

- Managing IBS requires some lifestyle changes such as cutting out certain foods, lowering your alcohol consumption, and increasing your exercise. But it's not as simple as saying that if all people cut out broccoli, for instance, then it will get better. Each person is unique, so finding out what triggers your IBS is essential. Do this by keeping a food diary and working out what seems to bring on a bout of IBS.

PROFESSIONAL HELP

- Your doctor would be the first person to see if you suspect you have IBS so they can rule out more serious conditions. An osteopath can then help alleviate symptoms of bloating, constipation, and gas by improving the function of the bowels. A dietician can also help you explore the root cause of your IBS.

- When I see a patient with IBS, I massage the surface of the stomach to stimulate the bowels into working again, while also manoeuvring any blockages through the intestines to the rectum so they can be expelled. At the same time, I also try to improve the lymphatic drainage and blood supply. Tension around the spine also needs to be released as the natural contractions of the bowel are controlled by the nerves, and if your lower back is tight this process might not work as well.

- Massage can really help with bloating, and clients often come with a full, bloated stomach and by the end their stomach is flat again. I've even had some clients with permanent bloating, who thought they were overweight and actually their rounded tummies were due to bloating, not weight gain, and were gone by the end of the session.

- If you can afford it, consider doing a food-intolerance test. You can do these privately and you can find out their cost on the provider's website. I have many clients who are athletes and eat really healthily, but they still have food intolerances and these tests have picked them up.

There have been some small, controlled studies in the US that support the effectiveness of osteopathic manipulative therapy in managing the symptoms of IBS. In one study 68 per cent of participants reported an improvement in their symptoms after receiving osteopathic treatment compared to 18 per cent who received conventional treatment.

CONSTIPATION

We all know that constipation is when you have difficulty passing stools as it's an incredibly common condition. I see clients of all ages with it, particularly pregnant women because of all the hormonal changes in their bodies. It is estimated that one in seven adults and one in three children suffer from constipation at any given time. Older clients are also more susceptible to constipation as they are not as active as they used to be, and this slows their metabolism.

The bowels are a smooth muscle that automatically contracts to push our food through, which normally takes between twenty-four and seventy-two hours. Everyone has a natural schedule for how often they need to go to the loo, and for a healthy person it can vary from three times a day to even once every couple of days. Constipation is when your personal schedule is knocked off course or if you haven't gone to the toilet for over three days. This usually means that there is a blockage of stools that can cause discomfort, bloating, and tiredness. When I'm bloated or constipated, I often get lower-back pain, which has nothing to do with the structure of the muscles, tendons, joints, or ligaments there. Instead, it's pressure from the bowels on the spine, and once the bloating is released then the pain goes with it.

Constipation often happens because of the food we eat, but I don't want to dive into the topic of nutrition – we all have a pretty clear idea of what we should and shouldn't be eating but, for various reasons, we don't always do this. What I do want to say, though, is that constipation should be treated in a similar way to pain. It's another message from our bodies that something isn't quite right and, in its more extreme forms, it can cause serious, sharp pains. I've had clients tell me that the pain was so bad they had to lie down on the bathroom floor. It's not something to be ignored.

We're all different and have differing guts and intolerances. Even the way our food circles through our intestines differs from person to person. You might have a wider section near your spine and your food collects there. In some cases, it can press on the spine causing pain, or even on the bladder, leading to an urgent need to pee. We all look different on the outside and, when it comes to how our intestines fold, we look different on the inside too. This is why stomach massage by an experienced professional can really help as they will be able to pinpoint where your specific problem area is.

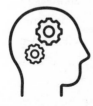 Start with your pain scale and **STOP**, and then consider the following:

- **S**ite: Lower part of the belly

- **T**ype: Pain can be an ache or cramps in the abdomen. You might also feel nausea and bloating.

- **O**nset: Symptoms usually last for a short time although they can be chronic in some cases, particularly during pregnancy and among the elderly.

- **P**rovoked by: Not eating enough fibre, not exercising enough, or not drinking enough water. Constipation has also been linked to stress and depression. Certain painkillers, such as codeine, can also cause constipation.

Stools can tell us so much about how our digestive system is working and what our body is lacking. There is even a medical chart that shows us what the appearance of our stools can mean (see Figure 10.2). Before you shudder at the idea of staring at the contents of your toilet bowl every day, let me say that it is a really good habit to get into and can act as a quick alert that something needs adjusting before you get into real problems.

FIG. 10.2
STOOL SHAPES AND WHAT THEY CAN TELL YOU

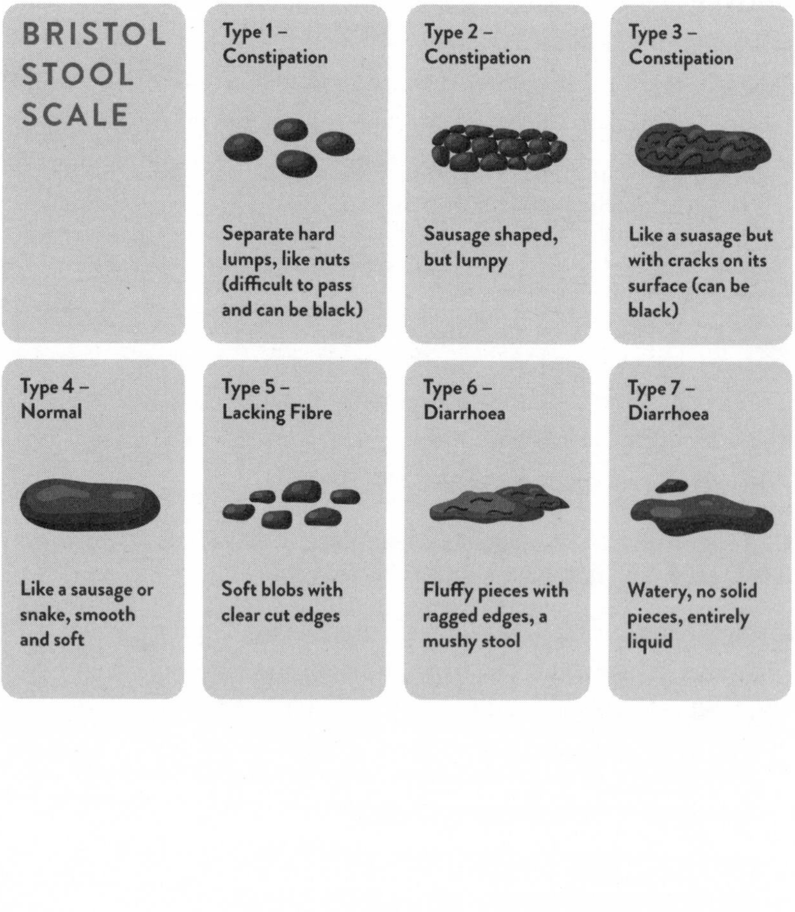

BRISTOL STOOL SCALE

Type 1 – Constipation

Separate hard lumps, like nuts (difficult to pass and can be black)

Type 2 – Constipation

Sausage shaped, but lumpy

Type 3 – Constipation

Like a suasage but with cracks on its surface (can be black)

Type 4 – Normal

Like a sausage or snake, smooth and soft

Type 5 – Lacking Fibre

Soft blobs with clear cut edges

Type 6 – Diarrhoea

Fluffy pieces with ragged edges, a mushy stool

Type 7 – Diarrhoea

Watery, no solid pieces, entirely liquid

- Constipation can be treated at home with some simple lifestyle changes such as drinking lots of water, getting more exercise, and introducing more fibre into your diet. Some foods with lots of fibre are beans, oats, berries, avocado, sweet potatoes, and broccoli.

- It is thought that probiotics can help ease the symptoms of IBS. You can buy yoghurts or drinks with these in, and they are thought to restore the balance of bacteria in your gut.

- If you can't afford a therapist, then try the self-massage technique at the end of the chapter.

PROFESSIONAL HELP

- An experienced osteopath can help loosen any compacted stools through massage. I always treat the back at the same appointment, as clients can be stiff in their mid-back and once this is loosened up, their bowel movements improve. Massage can help so much with constipation and bloated stomachs that there are therapists who specialize in massaging the stomach to move the food through, resulting in a flatter stomach.

- I am a big fan of colonics and there is more about them in Chapter 17 on alternative therapies.

If your constipation symptoms last for more than a few days it is a good idea to get them checked out by a doctor.

INDIGESTION AND ACID REFLUX

Indigestion describes pain and other symptoms felt in the top part of your abdomen, one of which is acid reflux (also known as heartburn). Acid reflux is when the acid from your stomach travels up your throat. It is often an accepted part of life by so many of my clients, including a lot of pregnant women. They reach for the antacids, the problem is dealt with for a couple of hours, but then it comes back again … and again. Like painkillers, antacids are a plaster and don't get to the root cause of the issue, which is often the diaphragm.

PATIENT FILES: INDIGESTION AND REFLUX

Stuart came to me with mid-back pain that he'd had for a few weeks. At his first appointment, he mentioned that acid reflux was starting to interfere with what he could eat, and that he had been using antacids for years. What he hadn't realized was that the two symptoms were linked. He had worked in an office for years, sitting at a desk all day, and his shoulders were rolled inwards. After I examined him, it was clear that the pain in his back was actually a referred pain from his stomach, which wasn't functioning very well. I worked on opening up his chest and diaphragm and the acid reflux reduced.

Most of us have heard of the diaphragm, but what exactly is it? The diaphragm is a sheet of muscle that is shaped like a parachute and sits just below your heart and lungs. It has two main roles: to separate the chest from the abdomen; and pull air into your lungs by contracting (see Figure 10.3). When viewed from above, you will see that there are three holes in the diaphragm to allow an artery and vein, large blood vessels and the tube that connects the stomach to the throat to pass through. The diaphragm is like any other muscle and can become tight. If it does, it can press on the tube that connects the stomach to the throat and force the acid up from the stomach. Because the diaphragm is a muscle, it can be treated by an osteopath to reduce any tension and lessen acid reflux.

What I often see in clients with acid reflux is that their shoulders are hunched inwards, and this change to their posture contributes to acid reflux. Opening up their chest works well to change their posture and sometimes this is the only thing they need to lessen their acid reflux.

FIG. 10.3
POSITION OF DIAPHRAGM IN BODY

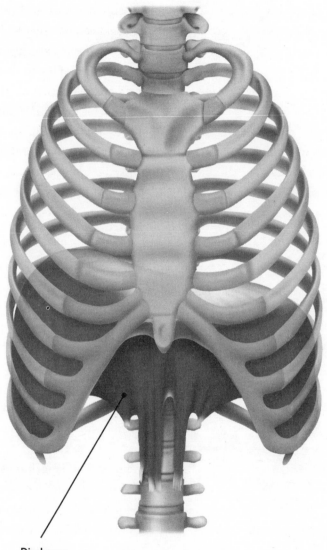

Diaphragm

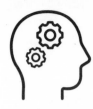

Start with your pain scale and **STOP**, and then consider the following:

- **S**ite: Upper abdominal area and throat.

- **T**ype: It can be a dull ache, uncomfortable fullness soon after starting eating, regurgitation of food, cramps in the stomach, a burning sensation in the chest, and the feeling of stomach acid travelling up your throat.

- **O**nset: Normally after eating, although it can be at any time, particularly with pregnant women.

- **P**rovoked by: Eating a heavy meal, overeating, eating too fast, eating spicy or fatty foods. It is also linked to drinking alcohol and can be provoked by exercising after eating, bending forwards, stress, and anxiety.

SELF-HELP

- Indigestion and acid reflux can often be helped with some simple lifestyle adjustments. Keep a food diary and avoid the food that is triggering your symptoms. The following are commonly known to provoke it: coffee, alcohol, chocolate, citrus fruit, and large meals. Sometimes painkillers can also make it worse.

- Lying down can make it worse, so try to remain upright after meals.

- People with acid reflux often breathe from their chest rather than their stomach. This makes their breaths shorter. It's good to practise breathing with your stomach rather than your chest, and there is more about this in Chapter 18 on stress.

- Osteopaths can work on improving the function of the stomach by working on the surrounding tissues, particularly the diaphragm, mid-spine, and oesophagus. I massage around the front of the neck to loosen up the muscles and to aid lymphatic drainage and blood flow. Acid reflux can often be because of poor posture, when people are hunched in on themselves, so working on opening up your chest can help. Massage around the stomach, diaphragm, and ribs also helps open up the chest.

OTHER COMMON ABDOMINAL CONDITIONS

- *Pain and bloating from the menstrual cycle* are things an osteopath can help with. Lymphatic drainage and visceral massage around the abdomen help with bloating. Loosening the muscles and some gentle mobilization around the lower back, buttocks and legs can help ease period pain.

- An *abdominal strain* is most common in athletes or people who play a lot of sport. These muscles are usually strained from a sudden twisting motion, too much exercise, or overused muscles. They should be treated in the same way as any other strained muscle.

- *Appendicitis* is a serious condition that can start as a mild cramping pain that comes and goes before gradually becoming much worse. I've had several clients come to me with clear signs of appendicitis and I've had to send them straight to hospital. The pain tends to be on the right side of the lower stomach or around the bellybutton. Appendicitis can be life-threatening and needs immediate medical attention.

- *Gallbladder inflammation* is discussed in more depth in Chapter 2, when a client came to me with pain in his shoulder caused by gallstones. Gallstones are very common and affect around one in ten people. They are often asymptomatic, but can cause pain. There can be serious complications from gallstones, so they need to be treated quickly if you are suffering from them.

- A *hernia* is when internal tissue from the abdomen pushes through a weak muscle or tissue wall. There will often be a lump, and it is more common in men than women. There are many types of hernia depending on what is poking through, such as your bowels or stomach, and where it is. You might require surgery to repair the muscle or tissue wall.

- *Crohn's disease* is inflammation of the digestive tract that causes severe pain and problems with drawing nutrients from food. There are no known cures, but medication and dietary changes can help manage it.

- *Ulcerative colitis* is a similar condition to Crohn's disease, but it only affects the colon rather than the entire digestive tract.

- *Coeliac disease* happens when the immune system attacks the small intestine when you eat gluten. It can cause pain, bloating, and diarrhoea. Dietary changes to cut out gluten are needed to treat it.

- Because of the number of visceral organs in the abdomen, there is a lot that can go wrong here. If you are feeling pain in your abdomen, then take a look at Figure 10.4, which explains which organ the pain might be linked to, and then book an appointment with your doctor.

FIG. 10.4
ABDOMINAL PAIN AND WHAT IT MIGHT MEAN

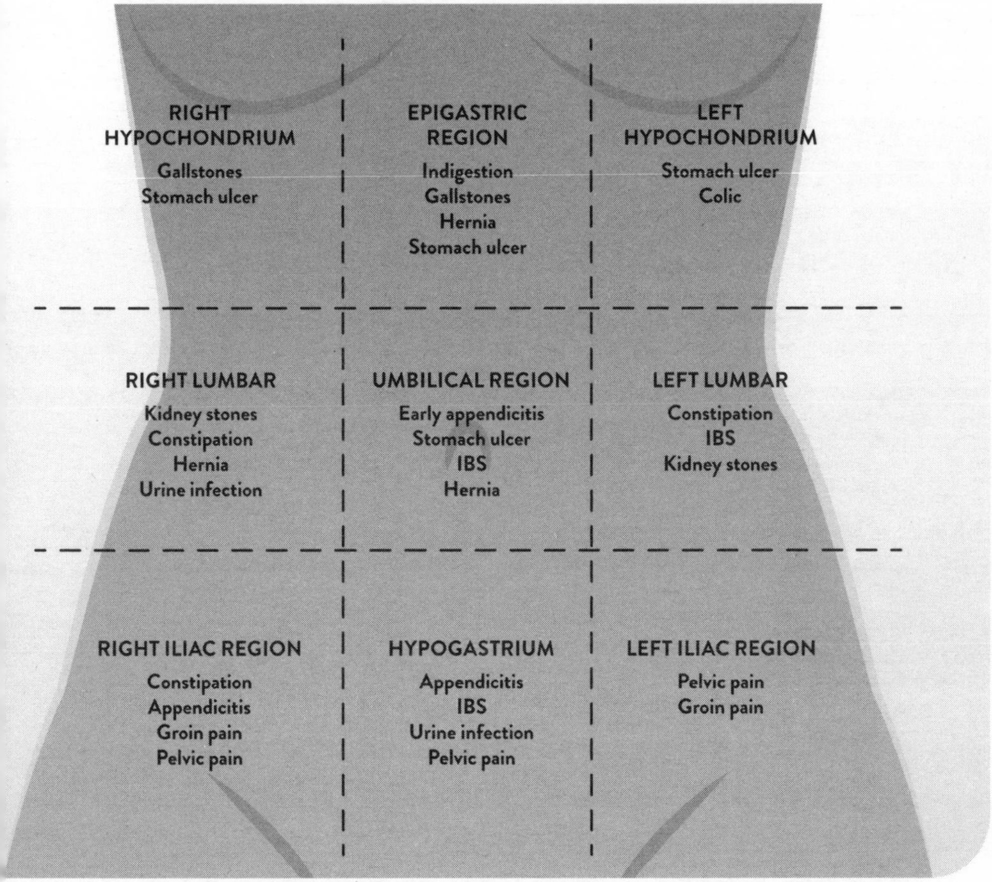

RIGHT HYPOCHONDRIUM

Gallstones
Stomach ulcer

EPIGASTRIC REGION

Indigestion
Gallstones
Hernia
Stomach ulcer

LEFT HYPOCHONDRIUM

Stomach ulcer
Colic

RIGHT LUMBAR

Kidney stones
Constipation
Hernia
Urine infection

UMBILICAL REGION

Early appendicitis
Stomach ulcer
IBS
Hernia

LEFT LUMBAR

Constipation
IBS
Kidney stones

RIGHT ILIAC REGION

Constipation
Appendicitis
Groin pain
Pelvic pain

HYPOGASTRIUM

Appendicitis
IBS
Urine infection
Pelvic pain

LEFT ILIAC REGION

Pelvic pain
Groin pain

You can check for certain types of hernias by placing your hand on the lump and then lying down. A common sign of a hernia is if the lump disappears or reduces in size. Another sign is if it gets bigger when you cough or sneeze.

STRETCHES AND EXERCISES FOR THE ABDOMEN

Massage around the stomach is very helpful for unblocking constipation, but before trying it you should check the warning flags listed earlier in this chapter, as it is not suitable if you have any of these signs.

Another area of our body that doesn't get enough attention is the pelvic floor muscles (see Figure 10.5). Strengthening these muscles can help with both incontinence and erectile dysfunction. They can also aid your recovery following pregnancy and have even been known to help with lower-back pain. As with all the exercises in the book, if they are painful or make your injury worse then please stop them immediately.

FIG. 10.5

PELVIC FLOOR MUSCLES

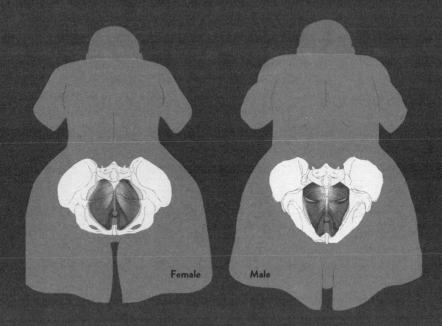

Female   Male

1

My favourite self-massaging technique for constipation is to lie on my back with my knees bent and feet flat down on the floor. With both your hands use your fingertips to massage your tummy in a circular motion. Do this firstly clockwise and then anticlockwise. When you do this, check for any areas that are tender and take a deep breath in and out, which can act as a release. Concentrate on massaging these tender areas by applying gentle pressure until they feel more relaxed.

2

Imagine that you're peeing (stick with me on this one) and then try and stop it mid-flow. Now imagine that you're about to pass wind and stop that from happening as well. The muscles you feel contracting in your groin are the pelvic floor muscles and holding this contraction for five to ten seconds will help strengthen them (see Fig. 10.5). Alternatively, you can do quick contractions and releases for five to ten seconds.

CHAPTER 11

Lower back

Two-thirds of my clients come to me because of back pain, and most of these cases are for pain in the lower back. It really is the epicentre for pain. In fact, 80 per cent of people will experience lower-back pain at some point in their life.

The reason that we have so many problems with our lower back is not because it was badly designed, it's because in our modern world we don't do the things our backs were designed for. Backs weren't meant to be stationary in a chair for eight hours a day. Instead, our bodies expect us to exercise for several hours each day, mostly walking and occasionally sprinting. Because we are so immobile, our muscles suffer deconditioning from lack of use, or are strained because we repeat the same action over and over again. Pain flares. We ignore it, because we don't have time to deal with anything else in our busy lives, and these early warning signs are missed, even though the clues are there. We carry on with a two, three or four on the pain scale, hoping it will just go away, but all the time the structures in our backs are gradually deteriorating until a pain rating of six, seven or eight rears its head.

But why does lack of movement damage our lower back specifically? Why not our shoulders or upper back? The main reason is that the lower back supports a huge amount of the body's weight, which

"
We don't do the
things our backs
were designed for.
"

presses down on it every day. Three of the vertebrae in the lower back take the brunt of the weight – that is, the L4 and L5 and S1 vertebrae at the base of the spine (see Figure 11.1). When we lift things, the lower back is also expected to compensate as we often forget to lift with our legs and engage the strong glutei muscles in our bums. The lower back is also far more mobile than the upper back, because it doesn't have several ribs strapped to it, so the lower back also helps our torso to twist, which again makes it vulnerable.

FIG. 11.1
VERTEBRAE OF THE BACK

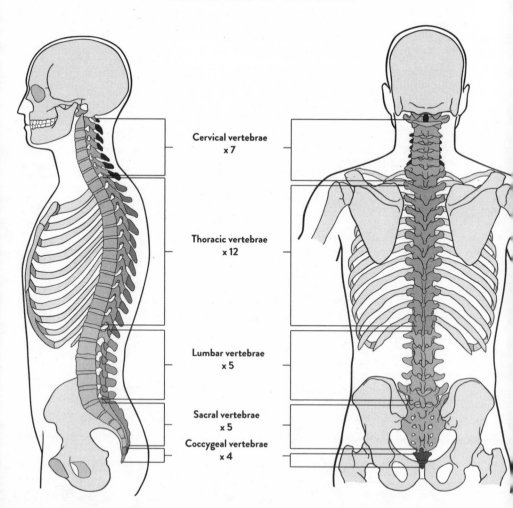

Cervical vertebrae
x 7

Thoracic vertebrae
x 12

Lumbar vertebrae
x 5

Sacral vertebrae
x 5

Coccygeal vertebrae
x 4

IS YOUR LOWER BACK HEALTHY?

Try the following slowly, so you don't wrench any of your muscles.
A healthy lower back should be able to do the following:

1
When you are seated, be able to lean backwards 45 degrees and not feel any pain.

2
When standing and keeping your legs straight, you should be able to lean down and ideally touch your toes. If you can't do this, then you should at least be able to reach your shins.

3
When standing up straight, bend your torso to the side. Your hands should be able to slide down the outside of your thighs to your knees. You should be able to do this on both sides.

4
Lastly, the lower back connects to your hips, which causes more potential complications. If your hips aren't working well, this puts more pressure on the lower back to compensate, so the muscles get tight and pull on the joints – everything is connected and any problems cause a domino effect.

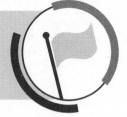

There are several warning flags when it comes to the lower back so always seek urgent medical attention if you experience any of the following:

- Severe lower-back pain, which is an eight or above on the pain scale

- Pain that is constant, where nothing alleviates it, including rest and painkillers

- Numbness or weakness in one or both legs

- Urinary or bowel incontinence or unusual changes

- Numbness or loss of feeling around the area that you would use to sit on the saddle of a bike

- Fall, trauma, or accident

- Previous history of cancer

- You are over the age of 50 with persistent lower-back pain

- No improvement after six weeks of treatment

- Unexplained weight loss

- Night pain that disturbs or stops you from sleeping

- History of HIV

- Recent TB diagnosis

- Lower-back pain combined with one or more of the following: frequent need to urinate (particularly at night), a painful burning sensation when urinating, difficulty starting to urinate or stopping it, erectile dysfunction, blood in urine or semen.

MOST COMMON LOWER-BACK CONDITIONS: MUSCLE STRAIN AND LIGAMENT SPRAIN

If you come to see me for any condition and are over the age of 25, I can guarantee that I will find tightness in the muscles in your lower back. There are lots of tiny muscles on each side of your spine that are often tight, along with the larger latissimus dorsi muscles (see Figure 11.2), which are closer to the surface. You might be asymptomatic, but these muscles will still need loosening. Over the years, I have learnt that even if someone comes to me with an ankle sprain, I still need to check their lower back and loosen any tension there as well.

Chronic, painful muscle strain in the lower back usually only happens to clients who have physically demanding jobs, or who do a lot of exercise. Clients with less demanding jobs will also strain their muscles but through inactivity. This may be a lower-level pain or asymptomatic, but the repercussions will occur later when the tightness impacts on another muscle or joint.

FIG. 11.2
MUSCLES OF THE LOWER BACK

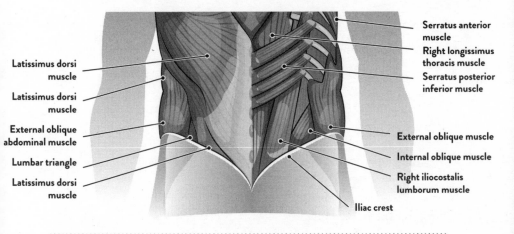

Latissimus dorsi muscle

Latissimus dorsi muscle

External oblique abdominal muscle

Lumbar triangle

Latissimus dorsi muscle

Serratus anterior muscle

Right longissimus thoracis muscle

Serratus posterior inferior muscle

External oblique muscle

Internal oblique muscle

Right iliocostalis lumborum muscle

Iliac crest

If you have read any of the chapters in this book on other areas of the body, then you will know that ligament sprains and muscle strains are rarely grouped together. But when it comes to the lower back, they have similar symptoms and treatment requirements.

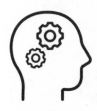

Start with your pain scale and **STOP**, and then consider the following:

- **S**ite: Across any area of the lower back.

- **T**ype: It can be a dull ache if it is a strain or sprain. If it is a rupture, it will be sharper. The area might be swollen or tender to touch.

- **O**nset: If it is sudden, it's likely that you will feel a popping or tearing sensation. It will also follow a sudden jarring or twisting movement, or after lifting something heavy. If it's gradual, it will come from overuse of the muscle or ligament, or from repeating the same movements.

- **P**rovoked: It will be made worse by any movement that contracts or stretches the muscle or ligament. You might have difficulty with walking or even standing.

SELF-HELP

- At home, you should try and rest the area if you can. **R**est, **I**ce, **C**ompression, and **E**levation always help if it is acute and inflamed (see page 70), or apply heat if there is no inflammation and the onset isn't recent.

- When I have strained back muscles, I like to have a hot bath with some Epsom salts sprinkled in. The heat from the water is therapeutic as it relaxes the muscles. There isn't much evidence that Epsom salts aid this process – they contain magnesium, which is an essential mineral we often lack, but there is no scientific evidence that this can be absorbed through the skin – yet I still like them. They're also cheap to buy and I know quite a few clients who also think they are beneficial. Placebo effect or not, I usually feel more relaxed and in less pain after using them.

- At home, stretching is also really helpful. Lie down on either your bed or the floor with your knees bent and feet on the mattress or floor (see Figure 11.3). Hold this position for several minutes. It may seem too simple to be of any use, but it's very beneficial for the muscles in the lower back. If you want to, you can then bring your knees up to your chest and hug them with both arms.

- For general muscle tightness, a cheap thing to buy is a softball (it's larger than a baseball and actually quite hard and I recommend them to all my clients over any other type of ball). Place it on the floor and lie on top of it with your knees bent. Use your legs to lift yourself off the floor and manoeuvre the ball across the muscles in your back and bum that are tight.

- If you can afford a massage gun, and have someone who will use it on you, they are very good for treating general strains in the lower back.

PROFESSIONAL HELP

- You can see an osteopath or chiropractor for a muscle strain or ligament sprain.

- I start by examining the client to find where the tension is and give a light massage over the area. I usually dry needle the area for both acute and chronic conditions. Often a muscle or ligament overstretches because there is a problem with a joint, which might need clicking back into place to restore the function in the spine. Once that is done, the overstretched muscle or ligament will have a chance to recover.

- If a joint does need to be put back into place, the tissues around it should be treated first to make them less tight, and mobilization should be tried before clicking. The joint should also be tested to see if there is a difficulty with twisting or other movements – if you go straight in and click, you're not finding out the full story behind what is happening in the back; you're just skipping to the last chapter. Also, if one joint is out of sync, it doesn't mean that the rest of them need clicking as well, as that can be damaging.

- If you have a lower-back issue you probably also have a problem with your glutei, which are the large muscles in your bum. I always massage these for a client with lower-back problems and they usually need firm pressure (an elbow works well!)

- In other areas of the body, a completely torn ligament will often require surgery, but this isn't usually the case with the lower back.

FIG. 11.3
LIE ON YOUR BED OR ON THE FLOOR
WITH YOUR KNEES BENT

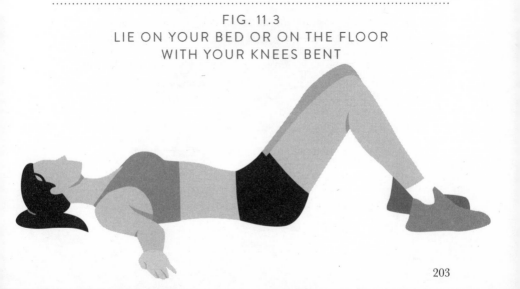

JOINT CONDITIONS

All along the spine are pairs of joints that link the vertebrae together, called 'facet joints' (see Figure 11.4). Most of the patients I see with facet-joint issues are over the age of 25, split equally between men and women. I first saw Emma after she had locked a joint when dancing at a party. She was in her late twenties and had twisted awkwardly to the side. Her muscle spasmed and her joint locked – it really is that easy to do.

These facet joints help with movement, but also stop us from twisting too far to the side. Like the entire lower back, these joints have a lot of pressure running through them, so they are susceptible to injuries and general wear and tear. When this happens, your joint is pushed out of sync and puts added pressure on your muscles.

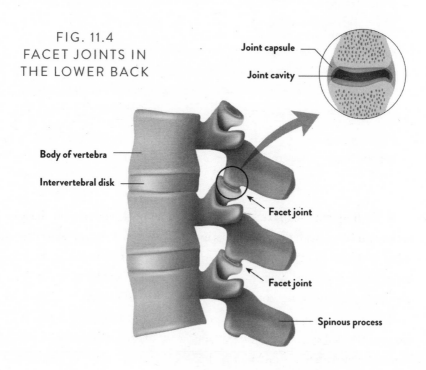

FIG. 11.4
FACET JOINTS IN
THE LOWER BACK

Joint capsule

Joint cavity

Body of vertebra

Intervertebral disk

Facet joint

Facet joint

Spinous process

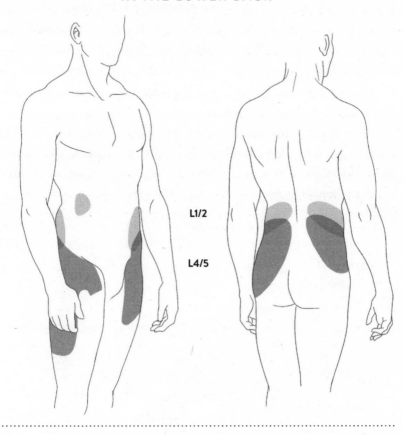

FIG. 11.5
REFERRED PAIN AND ITS ORIGIN
IN THE LOWER BACK

L1/2

L4/5

If you frequently lean backwards or twist your back, you're more likely to have problems with the facet joints in your lower back, but an issue can occur as the result of just one awkward movement. This is exactly what happened to my client, Vikram, when he was driving and he leaned right over to pick up the water bottle in the passenger seat footwell.

There is also the potential for referred pain from the facet joints in the lower back. So, you might feel pain in your hip that is actually a joint issue. As you can see from Figure 11.5, it's even possible to pinpoint which joint is affected just by the location of the referred pain.

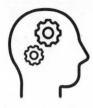

Start with your pain scale and **STOP**, and then consider the following:

- **S**ite: If the pain is localized it will be around the affected joint, and normally to one side rather than both sides. If the pain is referred, then it can travel to any of the shaded areas shown in Figure 11.5.

- **T**ype: It can be mild to severe pain. It will usually be a dull ache with stiffness, and then a sharper pain with movement or if you are in an awkward position. Many clients have described it as a 'catching' sensation when they move. In some cases, there can be nerve-root irritation, which will cause shooting pain down the leg, pins and needles, numbness, or weakness, but this is rare.

- **O**nset: This can be sudden or gradual. Clients often tell me that it started as a twinge in their back that lasted for months, or even for years, and rated around a two or three on the pain scale, and then it suddenly grew worse. If it's a gradual onset then it's usually due to wear and tear, rather than an injury.

- **P**rovoked: Joint conditions can be provoked by several things: leaning backwards, moving sideways, getting up from sitting, sudden movements, standing for long periods, and twisting movements. It is usually worse in the mornings or when a client goes from inactivity to activity.

> If you lean backwards with either a twisting motion or side bend and it brings on a sharp pain, it's likely that there is a joint condition. This test shouldn't be relied on alone as a diagnosis, but it's a good indication.

PROFESSIONAL HELP

- You can see either an osteopath or chiropractor for joint conditions.

- Firstly, the damaged joint must be located in the lower back and then the tissues around it should be massaged to loosen them up. The joint will then have to be pushed back into place through either mobilization or clicking. This is the only way the range of movement will be improved. Mobilization should always be tried first as there is less potential for damage compared to the more forceful method of clicking. As with all clicking, only the joint in question should be clicked unless there is a solid rationale behind clicking a higher or lower joint.

- The therapist then needs to investigate why this happened. It might be that, like the tiler in Chapter 2, you twist to the side a lot and so are shortening the muscles on one side and lengthening those on the other. If this is the case, then you need to stretch out the shortened side (the side you're turning towards). Daily stretches to help with this should prevent the injury from happening again; it's not the case that you have to spend lots of time in the gym lifting weights, trying to strengthen your lower back.

- If an osteopath or chiropractor can't provide you with suggested exercises and routines, then go to a physiotherapist, as they will be able to tailor a programme for your needs.

DISC CONDITIONS

Between each vertebra in your spine is a small disc that is about an inch wide and a quarter of an inch thick. There are twenty-three of them along the length of your spine, but it is the five in your lower back that are most vulnerable to damage, particularly L4 and L5 (discs are numbered L4, L5, etc., just as vertebrae are). Discs act as shock absorbers, prevent the vertebrae from grinding on each other, and allow a small amount of movement in your spine. They have a hard outer coating and inside is a jelly-like fluid. It is this jelly-like fluid that can leak if the disc is badly damaged (see Figure 11.6).

PATIENT FILES: DISC PROLAPSE

Miles had worked as a delivery driver for years, and for a long time he'd had a nagging lower-back pain that would come and go, normally getting worse at the end of the day. The pain was getting so bad when he was sitting in his van all day that he thought he was going to have to find a different job. After examining him, it was clear it was a disc issue and likely to be a prolapse. We came up with a plan to try and alleviate the pressure on his disc. For the next few weeks, I treated him regularly by applying traction to the area. At home, he didn't sit on his couch in the evening. Instead, he lay down on it with his legs raised on the arm of the sofa. He also changed the position of the seat in his van so it leaned further back. All of this helped take the pressure off the disc, so it was able to heal, and he could continue with his job.

As shown in Figure 11.7, leaking discs have different stages and obviously the severity of the bulge or rupture impacts on the pain and discomfort.

MYTH BUSTERS

Although we use the term 'slipped disc', the disc hasn't actually moved. Instead, what happens is that some of the jelly-type fluid inside the disc bulges out through the harder outer shell.

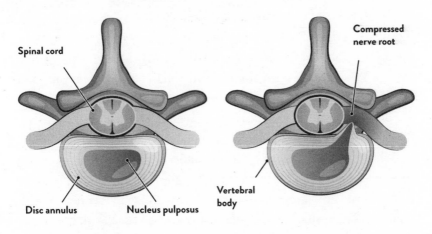

FIG. 11.6
NORMAL VS. LEAKY DISC

Spinal cord

Compressed
nerve root

Disc annulus

Nucleus pulposus

Vertebral
body

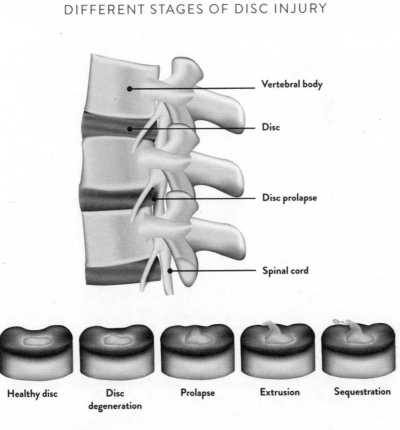

FIG. 11.7
DIFFERENT STAGES OF DISC INJURY

Vertebral body

Disc

Disc prolapse

Spinal cord

Healthy disc

Disc
degeneration

Prolapse

Extrusion

Sequestration

Disc degeneration is inevitable as we age, but it is increased by modern lifestyles. You might never have experienced pain in your lower back, but it's very likely that your discs are slowly being worn down if you don't lead an active lifestyle. As we age it is common for the discs to shrink and this is what leads to some elderly people getting shorter. When we are born, our discs are around 90 per cent water, but this slowly drops to 70 per cent as we age. Not drinking enough water can dehydrate your discs which causes them to lose their height, and can then lead to lower-back pain.

I don't often see people in their twenties with disc problems, unless they are athletes or have a history of serious weightlifting. The most common age group is people over 40, and I tend to see more men with these conditions than women, and the condition usually affects people who sit all day for their jobs, or perform repetitive actions throughout the day. By the age of 50, 90 per cent of us will have disc degeneration.

Disc conditions can affect the nerves as well but are not included here. Nerve-root irritation is discussed later in this chapter.

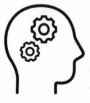 Start with your pain scale and **STOP**, and then consider the following:

- **S**ite: This depends on the level of the disc and whether there is referred pain. It can also be a localized pain to the disc in question.

- **T**ype: If there is no nerve-root irritation, it will be a dull ache, like a toothache. This can range from mild to severe pain.

- **O**nset: The pain will usually be sudden, even though the degeneration has been happening for a while. It can get worse throughout the day, and if the pain is acute then it can occur at night as well.

- **P**rovoked by: Coughing, sneezing, sitting for long periods, and bending forwards.

If you lean forwards and there is a sharp pain, it's likely there is a disc problem. This test shouldn't be relied on alone as a diagnosis, but it's a good indication.

SELF-HELP

- Traction, where the spine is gently separated, is really good for disc problems. You can do this at home with the help of a friend or family member. Lie on your back with the other person holding both of your ankles. They should then gently lean backwards, using their bodyweight to pull your legs towards them. This shouldn't be done too abruptly, or it can cause further irritation.

- Pilates is good for maintaining healthy discs as it's very effective at strengthening your core muscles.

- Rest is crucial for repairing a disc. If you can't sleep at night because of the pain, then the condition is serious and needs urgent medical attention.

PROFESSIONAL HELP

- You can see an osteopath or chiropractor for disc conditions. Your doctor might offer you a steroid injection and prescription painkillers.

- Clicking is not a suitable treatment for a joint with a disc problem and can make it worse. The only time this should be used is if one of the joints higher up or lower down from the disc in question is clicked.

- Dry needling is very useful for disc problems, and I use it on most of my clients who have this condition.

- There are many things you can do to help aid your recovery before deciding to have surgery. If I had this condition, I would try all of the above before deciding to go down the surgery route.

NERVE-ROOT IRRITATION

Disc conditions can have an added complication, when they press on a nerve. Sometimes, but not always, the change in the disc's shape can push on to a nerve causing a new set of symptoms. It's not just disc bulges that can cause nerve-root irritation in the lower back. Joint issues, outgrowths of bone, arthritis, inflammation, a spinal injury, infections, or an abnormal tissue growth can also cause nerve-root irritation.

PATIENT FILES: DISC PROLAPSE

Warren had been lifting boxes all day as he was moving house. He was in his mid-thirties and had hoped he could do it all by himself without needing to ask for any help. I saw him the following day after he'd woken up in the morning with a shooting pain going down his leg. He couldn't get out of bed and his wife had to help him to my clinic. Part of my assessment was to raise his leg when he was lying down – a shooting pain travelled right down his leg to his big toe. I looked at his big toe and it was weak. All of this pointed to a problem around the L5 vertebrae on his spine. I placed my hands on his L5 vertebra. It was very tender. We started with some traction and taking the pressure off the joint. This helped immediately. I examined him further and it was clear he had a disc pressing on a nerve, which was causing the shooting pain down his leg. I treated him regularly over the next three weeks and he made a full recovery.

With nerve-root irritation, there will usually be a referred pain to the lower parts of the body and possibly weakness, numbness, or pins and needles. Depending on where these symptoms are felt, you can even try to pinpoint which vertebra on the spine is near to the damaged nerve (see Figure 11.8). The key with nerve-root irritation is that the pain is usually worse in the limb than in the back.

Not all nerve pain in the lower back is 'sciatica'. I hear this term used a lot, but the sciatic nerve is only one of many that can be compressed and lead to pain.

FIG. 11.8
REFERRED PAIN LOCATIONS LINKED TO
THE LUMBAR AND SACRAL NERVES

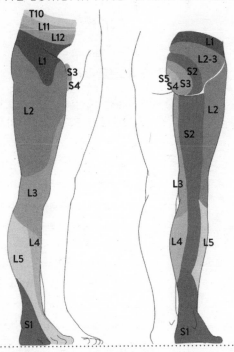

The sciatic nerve is probably the most well-known nerve in this area and most people have heard of sciatica. It is about the same size as your thumb (around 2cm) and is the largest nerve in the body. The sciatic nerve begins as five separate nerves when it exits the spinal cord in the lower back. It then merges into one in the bum before travelling down the length of the leg (see Figure 11.9). When people come to me with suspected sciatica, I always treat the piriformis muscle in the bum as the sciatic nerve can sometimes travel through the middle of it (see Figure 11.10). Often this becomes tight and compresses the sciatic nerve. Alternatively, the nerve can be compressed when it exits the vertebrae.

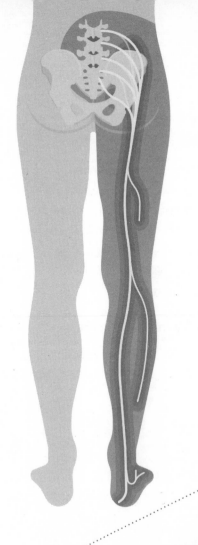

FIG. 11.9
SCIATIC NERVE

Lie on your back with your legs straight out and ask someone to lift each of your legs gently in turn. If there is a shooting pain down the leg, then it is likely you have nerve-root irritation in the lower back.

FIG. 11.10
SCIATIC NERVE AND
PIRIFORMIS MUSCLE

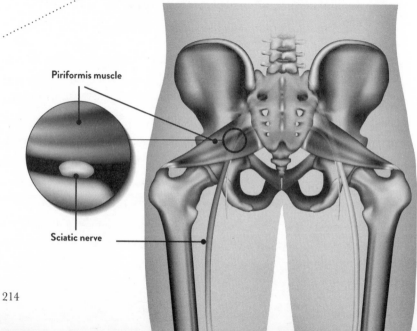

Piriformis muscle

Sciatic nerve

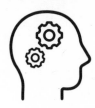

Start with your pain scale and **STOP**, and then consider the following:

- **S**ite: A referred pain that can be anywhere in the lower limbs, but is most commonly felt in the buttock, back of the thigh, or calf.

- **T**ype: There will be sharp shooting pains that can range from mild to severe. The pain is generally worse in the lower limb than in the back. There may also be numbness, pins and needles, tingling sensations, and some weakness in the leg. There can also be difficulty in walking if there is a weakness in one or both feet.

- **O**nset: Can be sudden or gradual.

- **P**rovoked by: Bending forwards, coughing, sneezing, laughing, sitting for long periods.

SELF-HELP

- Ice placed on the site of the pain can help take the edge off and reduce any inflammation.

- The best thing for nerve-root irritation is rest. If you can do this with your legs raised up on the arm of the sofa, it will take even more pressure off your lower back.

PROFESSIONAL HELP

- You can see an osteopath or chiropractor for nerve-root irritation.

- Treatment depends on where the nerve is compressed. If it is a joint issue, then mobilization or possibly clicking might be needed to manoeuvre the joint back into place. If it is a disc bulge, then traction is really beneficial. Both conditions are helped by mobilization to try and open up the area to take away the pressure on the nerve. Or, if it's a tight muscle pressing on the nerve, massage can help loosen up that tightness.

- Dry needling and cold laser therapy can also help alleviate pain, particularly if the area is very tender.

SACROILIAC JOINT PAIN

Where the spine meets the pelvis there are two sacroiliac (SI) joints, and joint pain here is very common (see Figure 11.11). This is particularly the case during pregnancy because these joints must loosen to make childbirth possible. As the pregnancy proceeds, the ligaments relax and the joint isn't held together as well. In addition to this, there is also the weight of the baby pushing down on them.

PATIENT FILES: SI JOINT

Nadia had started working for herself as a taxi driver. She'd just bought a new car and as she was getting out of it, she misjudged her step and landed heavily on her right foot. She felt the force of the misstep sweep up her leg and a sudden pain. She carried on with her day, but began to feel pain in her lower back on one side when she got in and out of her taxi and climbed the stairs in her house. There was also a referred pain in her groin. When she came to see me, I realized her pelvis and SI joint was out of sync. I worked on the muscles surrounding them before clicking the pelvis back into place.

You don't have to be pregnant to have SI joint pain. It's also common when the hip isn't working well in conjunction with the lower back. The SI joints can then come out of alignment or there can be irritation if they rub against each other. This is never an isolated condition; there will also be a problem somewhere else, such as lengthened and shortened muscles, or an imbalance of the pelvis.

Referred pain is very common from the sacroiliac joints and is felt around the hips, outside of the top part of the thigh, and down the legs. For this reason, it can be difficult to distinguish from lower-back pain involving nerve-root irritation.

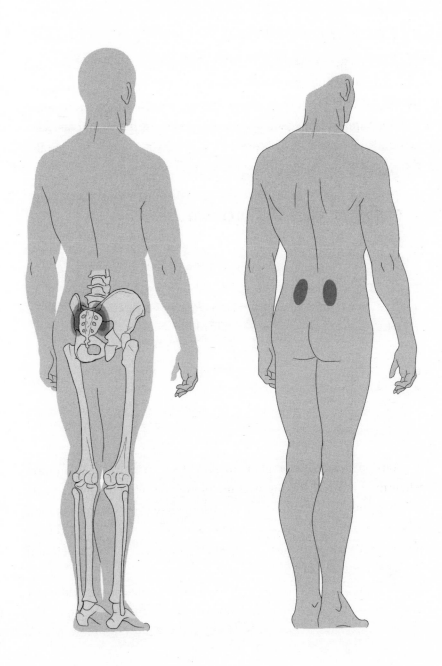

FIG. 11.11
LOCATION OF SACROILIAC JOINT

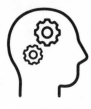 Start with your pain scale and **STOP**, and then consider the following:

- **S**ite: It is usually to the side of the spine, but the pain can also be referred to the bum, groin, and hip.

- **T**ype: It will be a dull ache when resting, and then a sharp/ stabbing pain when you move.

- **O**nset: It can be a sudden pain if there was a twisting movement or trauma. If the damage was caused by arthritis, then it will be gradual.

- **P**rovoked by: Going up and down stairs, getting out of a car, putting weight on the affected side, getting up from sitting, standing for long periods, and turning over in bed.

 A good test for this condition is standing on each of your legs in turn. If there is pain on one side of your back when you are hopping, it is likely to be from an issue with your sacroiliac joints.

SELF-HELP

- At home you can treat SI joint pain by placing a softball or tennis ball on the floor and lying on top of it. The ball should be placed on the surrounding areas to the SI joint rather than directly on the joint. Bend your legs to lift your body off the ground and use your legs to mobilize the ball to massage around the lower back. A massage gun also works well. There will normally also be issues with the lower vertebrae, so it's good to massage all around this area.

- You can see an osteopath or chiropractor for this condition.

- The joint needs to be put back into place through mobilization or clicking. At the same time, I massage the surrounding muscles to ease any tension there. As it is never an isolated condition, a therapist should also check your lower back, pelvis, and hip to try to work out where the source of the problem is.

OTHER COMMON LOWER BACK CONDITIONS

- Ankylosing spondylitis is an inflammatory disease that over time causes the vertebrae in the spine to fuse. It's more common in younger people and men. There is no cure but, with the right treatment, it's progress can be delayed.

- Spinal stenosis is when the gaps in the spinal cord narrow and put pressure on the nerves. In severe cases you might be offered surgery to relieve the pressure on the nerves.

STRETCHES AND EXERCISES FOR THE LOWER BACK

Simply lying on your back on the floor or a bed should help relieve the pain from most lower-back issues, but there are so many other simple exercises that you can do.

If you are in acute pain, you should reduce your pain levels through **R**est, **I**ce, **C**ompression, and **E**levation before trying the exercises (see page 70). When you feel ready to try them, start off slowly with minimal movements to check your body's reaction, as you don't want your back to seize up again. As with all the exercises in the book, if they are painful or make your injury worse then please stop them immediately.

1

Lie on your back with both knees bent and your feet on the floor. Use both hands to lift one knee towards your chest and hold it there for a few seconds. Do the same with the other knee.

2

Lie on your back with both knees bent and your feet on the floor. Place your arms on the floor with your palms facing down. Gently rock your knees from side to side for a few minutes.

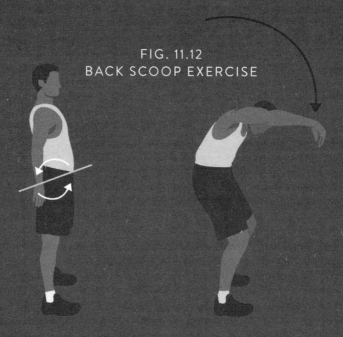

FIG. 11.12
BACK SCOOP EXERCISE

3

A good stretch for the quadratus lumborum (QL) muscles, which are on both sides of your lower spine, is the classic side stretch that we all did in school. These muscles are often strained so it's a great exercise for anyone with lower-back problems. While standing, place your feet wide apart. With one arm, reach your hand up and over your head. Lean to the side. Do the same with the other arm.

4

Place your feet shoulder-width apart and dip into a slight squat with your pelvis tilted backwards. Bring both arms down from your head to about shoulder height in a scooped shape (see Figure 11.12). You should feel a stretch in your lower back.

5

The next exercise is really good for disc problems and acute back pain, when you just need some relief from it. Lie on your back on the floor with your calves resting on a chair or stool. Your knees should be bent at a 90-degree angle (see Figure 11.13). Place your arms to the side. Take a deep breath and allow your back to relax.

6

The Child's Pose in yoga is very good at stretching your back muscles and taking pressure off the spine. From a kneeling position, sit back on your feet and lower your body so your head is close to the floor in front of your knees. Stretch out your arms in front of your head (see Figure 11.14). Keep your neck in a relaxed position and your head facing the floor. Hold the position for around twenty seconds.

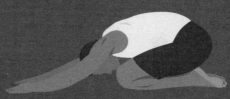

FIG. 11.14
CHILD'S POSE

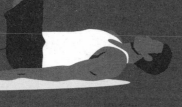

FIG. 11.13
EXERCISE FOR ACUTE
BACK PAIN

7

Lie on your back with both knees bent and feet on the floor. Take one of your legs with both arms and cross it over the other leg so your knee is positioned above your abdomen. With both hands gently pull this knee towards your opposite shoulder (see Figure 11.5). Do this on the other side as well. You should feel a stretch in your buttock.

FIG. 11.15
BUTTOCK
STRETCH

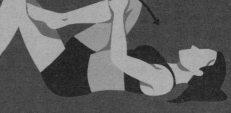

CHAPTER 12

Hip

Compared to the shoulder, the hip is an incredibly stable joint, owing to the strong ligaments that surround it. All this stability doesn't decrease the hip's mobility – considering there is only a single joint, we still enjoy a wide range of movement in a healthy hip.

SYMPTOMS CHECK

ARE YOUR HIPS HEALTHY?

When standing and placing an arm on a wall to support yourself, if you have healthy hips you should be able to:

1
Bend your knee up towards your chest.

2
Keeping your leg straight, lift your leg to the side and away from your body. You should be able to lift it more than 45 degrees and bring it back to your body without feeling any pain.

3
Swing your leg backwards and forwards with your knee straight and not feel any pain.

4
Move your feet inwards and outwards.

5
Walk backwards without any pain.

"

Considering there is only a single joint we enjoy a wide range of movement in a healthy hip.

"

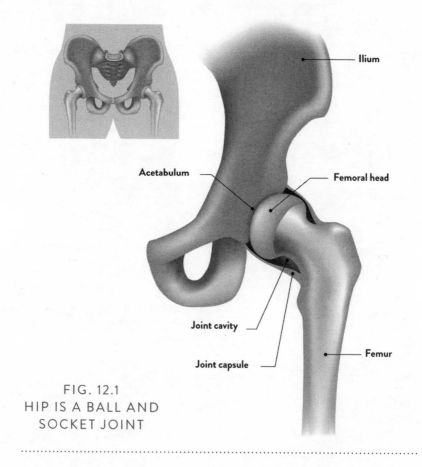

Acetabulum

Femoral head

Ilium

Joint cavity

Joint capsule

Femur

FIG. 12.1
HIP IS A BALL AND
SOCKET JOINT

The hip is a ball and socket joint that supports the weight of our body while also allowing us to walk and run (see Figure 12.1). Our hips expect us to walk regularly and many of the problems that occur there are because we aren't active. Consequently, there can often be added problems in the lower back and knees. The hip therefore needs to be treated holistically, so a therapist should examine the knees and lower back as well.

The hip is also an area to which pain is referred. When I see someone with hip pain it's often referred pain from the lower back or knee, so take a look at Chapters 11 and 13 as well, when considering hip pain. Since there is so much referred pain in the hip, it's a good idea to test whether the pain you are feeling is actually because of your hip joints and muscles. See the next page for a test you can do (Fig. 12.2).

When most people point to their hip they tap the side of their body, just below their waist, but this isn't where the hip joint is. It's actually in the groin and the socket is just above where your thigh starts.

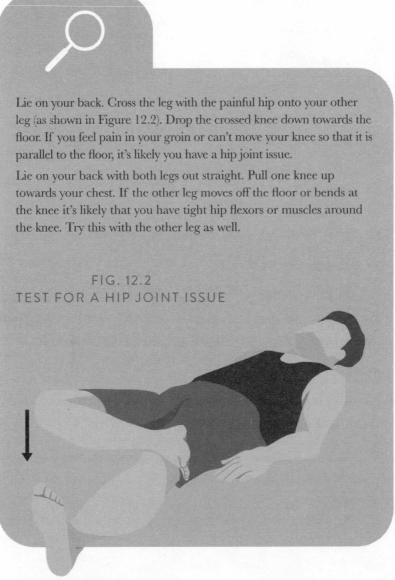

Lie on your back. Cross the leg with the painful hip onto your other leg (as shown in Figure 12.2). Drop the crossed knee down towards the floor. If you feel pain in your groin or can't move your knee so that it is parallel to the floor, it's likely you have a hip joint issue.

Lie on your back with both legs out straight. Pull one knee up towards your chest. If the other leg moves off the floor or bends at the knee it's likely that you have tight hip flexors or muscles around the knee. Try this with the other leg as well.

FIG. 12.2
TEST FOR A HIP JOINT ISSUE

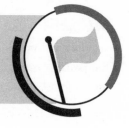

There are several warning flags when it comes to the hips so always seek urgent medical attention if you experience any of the following:

- New lump or bump in the groin or side of the hip
- Swelling
- Pain at night that is stopping you from sleeping
- History of cancer
- History of trauma
- Change in the hip's shape
- Unexplained weight loss
- A deep intense pain
- Constant pain that isn't alleviated by rest or painkillers
- Inability to walk

MOST COMMON HIP CONDITIONS: OSTEOARTHRITIS

Osteoarthritis generally affects older people, particularly if you have a job that requires repetitive actions or you are sedentary throughout the day. Surprisingly, it can also occur in younger people and I've seen several clients in their early thirties with hip osteoarthritis, particularly if they broke their hip bone when they were younger. Osteoarthritis in the hip is generally due to wear and tear and degeneration of the cartilage in the hip. Cartilage is a flexible tissue that covers all the joints in the body. It stops the bones from rubbing when they move over each other and is also a shock absorber. If the cartilage wears away it exposes the bones inside the hip joint and they will then rub on each other, causing damage to the bone.

The reason that the hips are so susceptible to osteoarthritis is because over the years there is a lot of pressure bearing down on them as they support the weight of the upper body. This is why the condition mostly happens in people over the age of 50. For more about osteoarthritis, take a look at Chapter 3.

PATIENT FILES: OSTEOARTHRITIS

Brian, a retired IT consultant, was in his late sixties when he first came to see me. He was waking up with stiffness in his hip every morning and it would usually take fifteen minutes for him to be able to walk normally again. I suspected osteoarthritis and this was confirmed when he went for an X-ray. He began a daily programme of stretching and also came to see me for treatment once a month. He went from never having stretched since his school days to stretching every day and actually enjoying it. His symptoms have now improved.

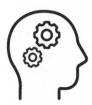

Start with your pain scale and **STOP**, and then consider the following:

- **S**ite: Front and outside of the hip, groin, and thigh. It can sometimes radiate down to the knee.

- **T**ype: It will be a dull ache, but there can also be a sharp or stabbing pain on movement. The hip can also feel stiff or even lock.

- **O**nset: It will be gradual and over time it will get worse. As the osteoarthritis progresses you may feel that one leg is shorter than the other.

- **P**rovoked by: Exercise, putting on shoes and socks, walking, getting up from a chair, or sitting for long periods. The hip will usually be stiff first thing in the morning for less than thirty minutes and then get worse at the end of the day.

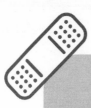

- Rest is only good for the hip in small amounts. Long term, the hip needs to stay active so that the stiffness doesn't get worse.

PROFESSIONAL HELP

- You can see an osteopath or chiropractor for treatment, and a physiotherapist can help with a programme of exercises.

- Firstly, a therapist will need to check the range of movement and see how much it has reduced. The aim is to bring back more movement through a combination of gentle mobilization and massage without aggravating the joint. I mainly use my hands when treating this condition to loosen up the muscles around the hips, lower back, and knee. Gentle traction can help relieve the pressure on the joint.

- Dry needling can also be effective in relieving pain.

- Tecar therapy is very good for osteoarthritis in the hip.

- If the progress of the osteoarthritis is advanced, then a walking stick might be needed, as well as orthotics if one leg is shorter than the other. These can be organized through the NHS or privately. Orthotics are a general term for prescription aids that help with recovery or assist people with a life-long condition. Examples of orthotics are insoles, splints, and callipers.

- Hip replacements are incredibly common once the cartilage in the hip joint has worn down. In the UK there are 80,000 hip-replacement procedures a year. Personally, I would only have a hip replacement as a last resort and I'd postpone the need for one by staying as active as possible, losing weight if advised to, and finding a therapist who can treat the surrounding tissues of the hip joint; and I would also include strengthening exercises in my daily routine.

IMPINGEMENT

If you've read Chapter 6 on the shoulder, then you'll know that a shoulder impingement usually occurs when a tissue gets trapped or catches on the joint socket. A hip impingement is slightly different because it occurs when the ball of the hip joint doesn't move smoothly against the cup of the joint. This happens for two main reasons: either the ball or the cup is slightly misshapen (see Figure 12.3).

A hip impingement is a common injury that can often have no symptoms for years. Despite this, it needs to be dealt with as it is a leading

FIG. 12.3
TYPES OF HIP IMPINGEMENT

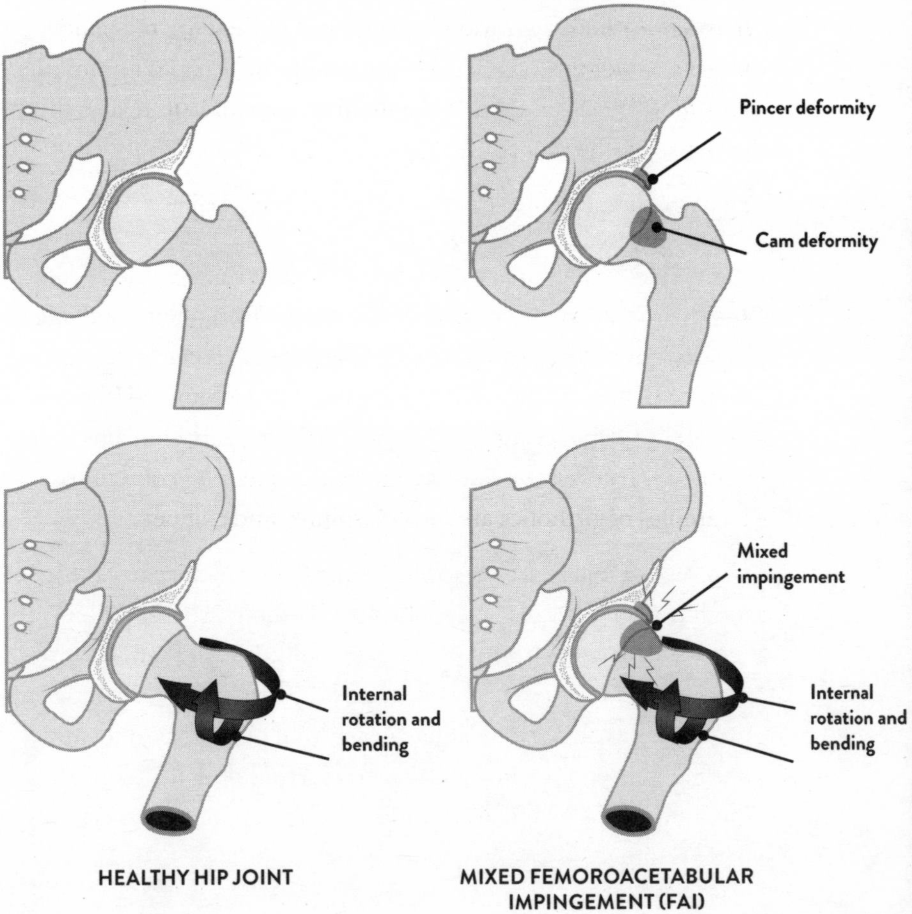

Pincer deformity

Cam deformity

Mixed impingement

Internal rotation and bending

Internal rotation and bending

HEALTHY HIP JOINT

MIXED FEMOROACETABULAR IMPINGEMENT (FAI)

PATIENT FILES: IMPINGEMENT

When I first met my client, Ashley, he had torn his quad muscle and needed treatment for this. As part of my examination, I tested for an impingement and it was clear that there was one. Ashley played football every weekend and felt stiffness in his hip whenever he kicked the ball. The impingement was the root cause of the problem, and the torn quad was the result.

cause of osteoarthritis. Hip impingements are really common among young sportspeople, particularly footballers, when they are teenagers or young adults. I have an impinged hip on my left side that I've had since I was a teenager. It's something that will never be completely cured, but I keep all the muscles around the hip loose and this improves my range of movement. If these muscles are functioning well, then the impinged hip won't impact on other areas of the body such as the lower back.

Clients rarely come to me because of a hip impingement because most people are unaware that they have one. Instead, they want treatment for lower-back pain, or a groin or thigh muscle tear. Because a hip impingement can be without symptoms for many years, and can be difficult to detect, it's a good idea to test for it first.

A quick way of checking if you have an impinged hip is to start by sitting down. Move the leg that is on the same side of the hip you want to test and rest your ankle on the lower part of the thigh of the other leg. If this is difficult to do or there is a catching sensation, it is likely you have an impinged hip.

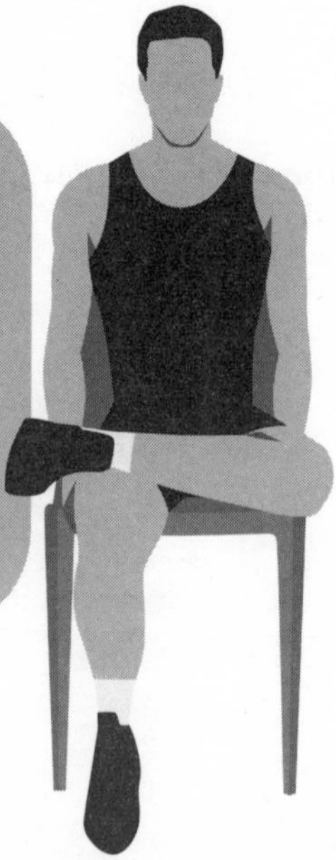

FIG. 12.4
TEST FOR A HIP IMPINGEMENT

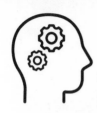

Start with your pain scale and **STOP**, and then consider the following:

- **S**ite: Groin or outer hip.

- **T**ype: A dull ache, catching sensation or a feeling that the movement in the hip is limited. The hip might also click. There can be stiffness if the condition worsens.

- **O**nset: Gradual and insidious – it is often without symptoms, but damage is still being done to the joint.

- **P**rovoked by: Sitting for long periods of time, moving the leg forwards, rotation of the hip.

SELF-HELP

- At home you can use a massage gun on the lower back and the muscles surrounding the hip. Be careful not to use it directly on the hip bone.

- Stretching is very important for a hip impingement. If you can keep the muscles around the hip working well, then there will be less complications from the impingement.

PROFESSIONAL HELP

- An osteopath will try and improve the range of motion in the hip.

- My aim with a hip impingement is to loosen the muscles around the hip and lower back to improve the movement in the hip. I use a combination of massage, gentle mobilization, and stretching.

- Dry needling and Tecar therapy work well on a hip impingement.

- If the stiffness and pain gets worse, you could have surgery. Several of my clients have had successful surgery that has improved the condition.

MUSCLE/TENDON STRAIN OR TEAR

There are over twenty muscles around the hip that can become tight and limit the movement in the hip joint. If you suspect that you might have strained a muscle or tendon in this area then look back at Chapter 3, which will help you decide whether it is a strain or a tear.

PATIENT FILES: MUSCLE TEAR

Sam booked an appointment with me four days after he felt a sudden pain when playing football. He'd had to stop playing in the middle of the game and thought that the pain would ease off over the next couple of days, but it didn't. When I examined him, there was bruising around his hip and it hurt when he used his hip flexor muscles. He was limping and rated the pain as a five on the pain scale. I suspected a tear to one of the muscles and he arranged an MRI scan, which confirmed a partial tear to the psoas muscle. I used Tecar therapy, and massaged and dry needled the area, all while avoiding stretching the damaged muscle.

The most common muscles to strain or tear are called the hip flexor muscles (see Figure 12.5). They are made up of several muscles and their job is to help bring your knee up towards your chest. These muscles can tear or strain because they are overworked or pulled beyond their normal range.

Another common muscle to strain is the tensor fasciae latae muscle (TFL), which is a muscle on the outside of the top of the thigh (see Figure 12.6). The TFL helps move the hip upwards and also rotate. It connects to the iliotibial (IT) band, which is a tendon that runs all the way down to your knee. There's more on the IT band in Chapter 13 on the knee.

FIG. 12.5
HIP FLEXOR
MUSCLES

FIG. 12.6
THE TFL MUSCLE
AND IT BAND

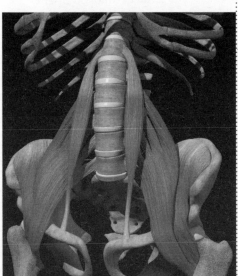

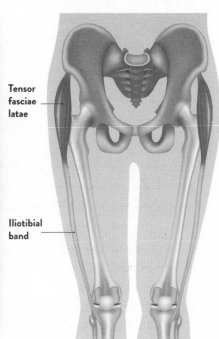

Tensor
fasciae
latae

Iliotibial
band

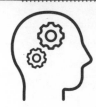 Start with your pain scale and **STOP**, and then consider
the following:

- **S**ite: Around the groin and front of the thigh.

- **T**ype: The initial pain can be sharp when you try to move your
  knee up to the chest or stretch the muscle. There can also be
  cramping, stiffness, swelling, and bruising. There might be some
  tenderness when pressed.

- **O**nset: Can develop gradually through overuse, or it can be
  sudden after changing speed or direction when running.

- **P**rovoked by: Running, kicking, or lunging. Walking or going up
  and down stairs might be difficult.

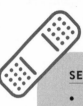

- **R**est, **I**ce, **C**ompression, and **E**levation are good for a recent tear or strain (see page 70). If the strain or tear isn't acute, and there's no inflammation, then you can try contrast bathing, where you switch between applying heat and cold to the area.

- You can use a massage gun at home, but be careful not to use it directly on the hip bone or on a tear that hasn't yet healed.

- A good exercise you can do at home is to kneel on a mat and then move one of your legs forward (as shown in Figure 12.7). Slowly lean forward until you feel a stretch through the groin. Do this on the other side as well. You can place a pillow underneath the knee that is taking your body weight if it is sore.

FIG. 12.7
GROIN STRETCH

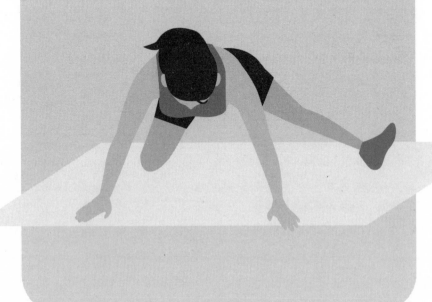

- You can see a physiotherapist, chiropractor or osteopath for this condition.

- The treatment depends on the severity of the strain or tear. Light massage around the area, rather than directly on the torn or strained muscle, is helpful, but should only be done by a skilled therapist as it can cause more damage or delay the healing process if there is a tear. Dry needling is usually beneficial, regardless of the grade of tear.

- In the days following the injury, I would just treat the tissue and then, once it is stable, I would start gently stretching the muscle. If it's a severe tear, then this would have to wait until there is further healing.

- If you can afford it, Tecar therapy helps repair soft tissue damage.

BURSITIS

All around our bodies there are 150 bursae that are normally situated near to a joint. These small fluid-filled pads are prone to inflammation, called bursitis, which is covered in Chapter 3. The bursa's job is to prevent tissue rubbing against other tissue or bone, but this means that they have a lot of friction running through them, which can lead to inflammation.

PATIENT FILES: BURSITIS

Aled was in his mid-forties and usually ran for miles every week until pain in his hip forced him to cut down his runs. He was surprised to learn that the pain in his hip wasn't one of the typical runner's injuries, but inflammation of the trochanteric bursa. For a while he had to rest and cut down on his training but, because he took this step, he made a full recovery.

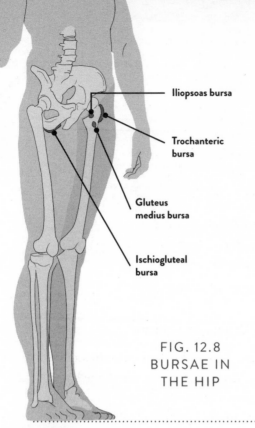

Iliopsoas bursa

Trochanteric bursa

Gluteus medius bursa

Ischiogluteal bursa

FIG. 12.8
BURSAE IN
THE HIP

Bursae can become inflamed because of a fall or repetitive movements. In the hip, the two most common bursae to become inflamed are the trochanteric bursa and the iliopsoas bursa (see Figure 12.8). In rarer cases bursitis can be caused by rheumatoid arthritis and gout.

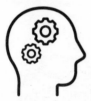

Start with your pain scale and **STOP**, and then consider the following:

- **S**ite: This depends on which bursa is inflamed. For the trochanteric bursa the pain will be on the outside of the thigh, and for the iliopsoas bursa it will be at the front of the hip and possibly be a referred pain to the buttock.

- **T**ype: Initially it can be sharp and intense. As time goes on, it will become a deep, dull ache. There can be accompanying stiffness and the pain might begin to spread down the thigh. There may also be swelling or tenderness, and it will usually be warm or hot to touch.

- **O**nset: It can be sudden or gradual.

- **P**rovoked by: Lying down on the affected side, getting up after sitting for a long period, squatting, walking, and getting out of a car. It can also be worse at night-time.

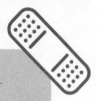

- Rest is essential for this condition as you don't want to move the joint too much and irritate it. If you can't rest it, because you still have to work, then try and fit in more breaks if you can.

- Anti-inflammatory painkillers, such as ibuprofen, can help in the short term.

PROFESSIONAL HELP

- You can see an experienced therapist for bursitis.

- The first thing to do is reduce the swelling and inflammation through massage. I would work away from the site of the bursa on the neighbouring muscles that might have caused the bursa to become irritated. I would use dry needling and cold laser therapy on the site of the bursa.

OTHER COMMON HIP CONDITIONS

- *Rheumatoid arthritis* is discussed more in Chapter 3, but the clearest sign of it is that it will affect both hips and the hip area will feel warm. It will usually start in the hands first before spreading to the hips. If there is stiffness in the joint in the morning, it will normally last for over an hour.

- A *labral tear* is when you tear the labrum cartilage around the rim of the hip's socket joint. This cartilage helps stabilize the joint and acts as a shock absorber. The pain can either be dull or sharp but will often be more painful when weight-bearing.

STRETCHES AND EXERCISES FOR THE HIPS

So many of the conditions we've talked about could have been prevented with some daily stretches to the hips. It really is an area for which ten minutes of your day can prevent so many problems when you reach middle age and reduce the impact of other conditions when you're elderly. So, if you can, try to find some time to stretch out those muscles around your hips.

As with all the exercises in the book, if they are painful or make your injury worse then please stop them immediately.

FIG. 12.9
LEG SWING EXERCISE

FIG. 12.10
SOLES OF FEET
TOGETHER EXERCISE

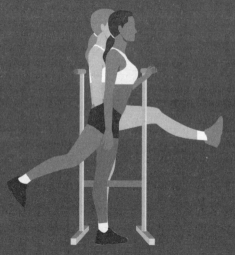

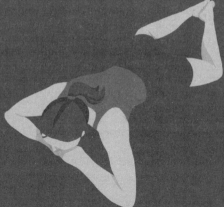

1

When standing, place one of your hands on a wall and gently swing your leg backwards and forwards. Turn to face the wall and swing the same leg from side to side (see Figure 12.9). Do this with your other leg as well.

2

Lie on your stomach and rest your chin on your hands. Bend your knees and allow the soles of your feet to meet. Gently press the soles of the feet together (see Figure 12.10) and you should feel a stretch in your buttocks and upper thighs.

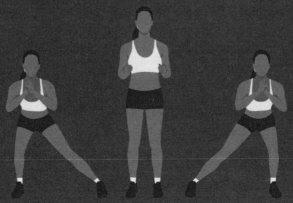

FIG. 12.11
SIDE GLIDE STRETCH

3

Start with a wide stance and hold your hands out in front of you. Bend one of your knees and shift your weight towards it until it is bent at 90 degrees and the other leg is straight. Gently raise yourself up again and then move your weight to the other knee and lower that one in the same way (see Figure 12.11). Do this five times on each side.

FIG. 12.12
WALL LEG ROTATIONS

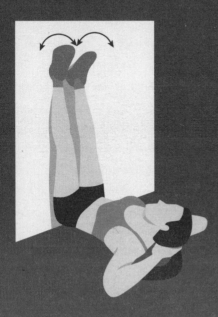

4

Lie on your back next to a wall. Raise your legs so they are vertical and lying flat against the wall. Rotate both of your legs inwards towards each other and then outwards (see Figure 12.12).

CHAPTER 13

Knee

I see clients of all ages with knee conditions. Those under 40 usually injure themselves because of a sudden twisting movement, often when playing sport. Those over 40 have normally damaged their knee through wear and tear and overuse. This usually happens because their knee has been slightly out of sync for years, creating accelerated damage to the joint.

The knee is the largest joint in the body and one of the most complex. Similar to the shoulder, it's not just one joint but three. It helps link the strong femur thigh bone with the two bones in the lower leg; the large tibia and slender fibula (see Figure 13.1). The knee is a modified hinge joint, which allows us to bend and straighten it. The joint also allows a small amount of rotation to the side, and when this is done too sharply, or too far, it can cause several acute injuries.

Many athletes and sportspeople, such as runners, have problems with their knees as so much force goes through them. Often, they don't warm up as well as they should, or they take up running after years of inactivity. If you are a keen runner, you will probably already know the basics of what you can do to protect your knees, but it's worth repeating: tarmac, uneven surfaces, and sharp turns around street corners all place added stress on our knees and should be minimized wherever possible.

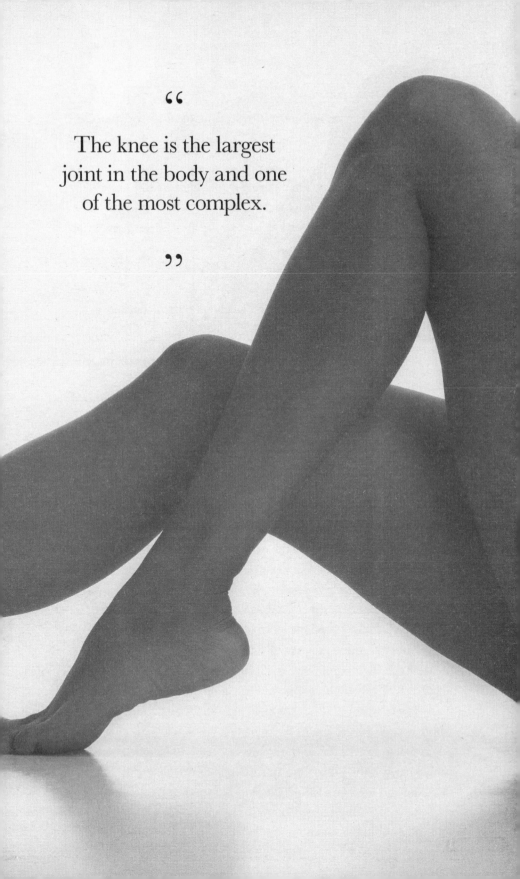

> The knee is the largest joint in the body and one of the most complex.

FIG. 13.1
ANATOMY OF THE KNEE

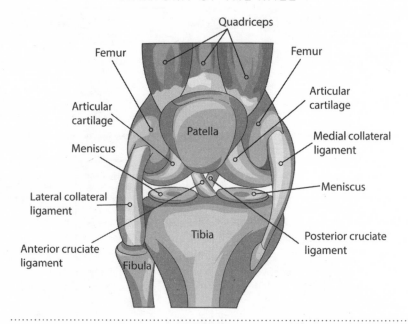

In my experience, knees are relatively easy to treat as the injuries usually arise from either a muscle imbalance in the quads, which are the large muscles at the front of the thighs, or from the popliteus muscle (see Figure 13.2), which is a small muscle at the back of the knee that helps stabilize it. The popliteus may be small, but it's very important as it helps us unlock the knee when we walk, as well as sit, stand, and rotate the knee. It is also used in the first stages of bending and when we fully straighten our knees. I find that with most knee issues there is a problem with the popliteus, and often it really does provide the key to restoring pain-free movement.

With all knee conditions, a therapist should treat the front, side, and back of the knee as they are all interconnected. Treating these areas often removes the tension in the knee and allows it to heal. Many people will resort to having their knees 'cleaned out' with an arthroscopy (a type of keyhole surgery used to diagnose and treat problems with the joints), but this doesn't deal with the root cause of the issue and therefore the problem is likely to return.

Knee conditions usually result from dysfunctions in the hips, lower back, or ankles. There can also be referred pain to the knee where the root cause is the hips, lower back, or ankles, so take a look at those other chapters as well.

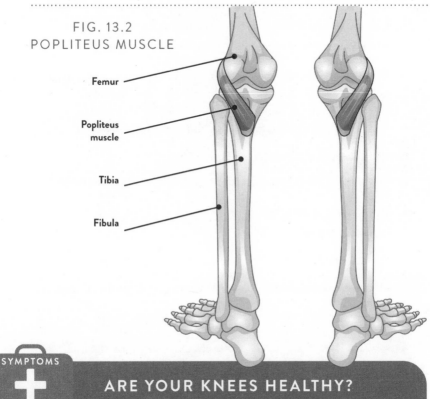

FIG. 13.2
POPLITEUS MUSCLE

Femur

Popliteus
muscle

Tibia

Fibula

SYMPTOMS

CHECK

ARE YOUR KNEES HEALTHY?

Healthy knees should be able to:

1
Bend and straighten fully.

2
Allow you to squat with no pain.

3
Allow you to squat with one leg and no pain.

4
Both knees should look the same, be the same size and not point inwards (use a mirror for this).

5
There shouldn't be any fluid or swelling around the knee.

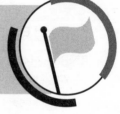

There are several warning flags when it comes to the knees so always seek urgent medical attention if you experience any of the following:

- Continuous pain that is present throughout the night, even when you rest the knee and take painkillers

- Any traumatic impact to the knee

- A fall

- If you can't straighten your knee and feel that it is locked

- If the knee feels unstable and gives way

- Difficulty with weight-bearing

- A new lump or an existing lump around the knee that increases in size

- Previous history of cancer

- Unexplained weight loss

- Recent surgery after which the swelling has increased

MOST COMMON KNEE CONDITIONS: PATELLOFEMORAL SYNDROME

Patellofemoral syndrome is the name for generalized pain at the front of the knee or around the kneecap. It's also known as 'runner's knee' although, like golfer's elbow, you don't have to be a runner to suffer from it. It's caused by overworking the muscles surrounding the knee, which impacts on the tendon going into the top joint of the knee. It's generally seen in younger people who are active.

In my experience, with 95 per cent of cases, the imbalance in the surrounding muscles is in the quads. These are the four muscles at the front of the thigh that share a tendon which goes into the top of the kneecap. Once these have been loosened, the pain will begin to lessen.

PATIENT FILES: PATELLA

Bo had been doing squats for years as part of his exercise routine. After he finished working out one day, he noticed an ache at the front of his knee. He tested the knee and couldn't fully bend it. He called me and I said it was likely that his quad muscles were overworked and he should try using a massage gun on them. He did this for ten minutes, which released the tension in the patella tendon, and the pain went away – one of my quickest patient recoveries.

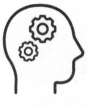

Start with your pain scale and **STOP**, and then consider the following:

- **S**ite: At the front of the knee, on or around the kneecap, behind the knee.

- **T**ype: A dull ache. The kneecap is usually tender to touch and there might be a clicking noise around the kneecap.

- **O**nset: Gradual and can get worse if you increase your activity.

- **P**rovoked by: Sitting with the knee bent, going up and down stairs, squatting.

Relax your knee so it isn't completely straight (if it's fully straight you won't be able to move your kneecap). Try to move the kneecap gently with your fingertips. If this doesn't hurt, then it's a good sign that you don't have patellofemoral syndrome.

Use your finger to tap on the kneecap and also above and below it. If you don't feel any pain, then it is unlikely that you have patellofemoral syndrome.

- **R**est, **I**ce, **C**ompression, and **E**levation are always useful if the area is acute or inflamed (see page 70).

- Using a massage gun on the quads can often help relieve this condition.

- If the vastus medialis obliques (one of the four muscles that make up the quads; see Figure 13.3) are weak or dysfunctional it can lead to stability issues and a change in the position of the kneecap that can make the knee vulnerable to injuries. To build strength there, I often advise clients to invest in a transcutaneous electrical nerve stimulation (TENS) machine.

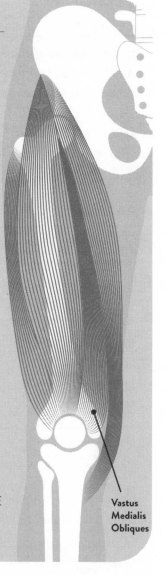

FIG. 13.3
POSITION OF VASTUS
MEDIALIS OBLIQUES MUSCLE

Vastus
Medialis
Obliques

PROFESSIONAL HELP

- You can see either a physiotherapist, chiropractor or osteopath.

- When treating this condition, I start by massaging and dry needling the quads. If the knee is too tender to touch, then I use cold laser therapy.

LIGAMENTS

Lots of ligaments are needed around the knee because there are so many bones to stabilize. I see all kinds of clients with damaged ligaments, but the one thing they all have in common is that this issue is usually preceded by a muscle imbalance in the knee that makes it vulnerable. Then there will be a sudden injury, from either a traumatic event, a twisting movement, or too much force going through the knee, and this is what damages the ligament.

> ### PATIENT FILES: LIGAMENT
>
> Charlotte was 17 years old and played a lot of netball at school. In the middle of a game, she caught a ball and rotated her body while her foot stayed still on the ground. She heard a pop in her knee and so did one of her teammates. She tried to carry on playing but her knee felt weak, as if it couldn't support her weight. When she sat down, her knee suddenly became very swollen. She came to see me a couple of days later and after examining her I thought she had torn her anterior cruciate ligament (ACL). This was later confirmed by an MRI scan. I treated Charlotte in stages, starting with massage after her surgery and then providing a rehabilitation plan so she could return to playing netball.

Our knees have four main ligaments that can become strained, partially torn, or completely torn (see Figure 13.1). These are:

- ACL: anterior cruciate ligament

- PCL: posterior cruciate ligament

- LCL: lateral collateral ligament

- MCL: medial collateral ligament

You can find more information on ligaments, sprains, and tears in Chapter 3, but in this chapter, I deal with each of the ligaments separately so you can try to identify which one has been damaged.

ANTERIOR CRUCIATE LIGAMENT (ACL)

This ligament is small compared to the other ligaments in the knee, but it has the crucial role of holding the femur to the tibia. It also stops the tibia from slipping forward and brings stability to the knee when it rotates. It's the ligament that is damaged most often in the knee.

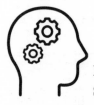

For ACL sprains or tears, start with your pain scale and **STOP** and then consider the following:

- **S**ite: Deep pain in the centre of the knee.

- **T**ype: Severe pain that will be sharp when you first injure it. This will be replaced by a deep ache with accompanying swelling. There will often be a feeling that the knee is about to give way. It will feel unstable and there will be a loss of movement.

- **O**nset: Sudden, usually after a quick change in direction or jumping and landing the wrong way or after a forceful impact to the knee.

- **P**rovoked by: Discomfort when walking, standing, putting pressure on the affected side.

POSTERIOR CRUCIATE LIGAMENT (PCL)

The PCL connects the femur to the back of the tibia and is a small ligament deep inside the knee, next to the ACL. It is much less common to tear the PCL than the ACL as it is less vulnerable. It is therefore normally only injured in contact sports or trauma, such as a road-traffic accident where the lower leg hits the dashboard. If you do tear your PCL, then it's likely you will have torn one or more of the other ligaments as well. When the other ligaments in the knee tear, there is usually a popping sound, but this isn't always the case with the PCL.

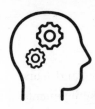

For PCL sprains or tears, start with your pain scale and **STOP** and then consider the following:

- **S**ite: Back of the knee.

- **T**ype: Sharp, deep pain but can also be a dull ache. It might swell and there will usually be stiffness in the knee. The back of the knee might be warm to touch. There might also be tingling or numbness if the tear is severe.

- **O**nset: It will be a sudden pain.

- **P**rovoked: Discomfort when walking, standing, putting pressure on the affected side.

LATERAL COLLATERAL LIGAMENT (LCL)

The LCL is a long ligament on the outside of the knee. Its job is to stabilize the knee and stop it from moving too far to the side. It connects the femur in the thigh to the slender fibula bone in the lower leg.

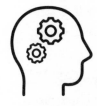

For LCL sprains or tears, start with your pain scale and **STOP** and then consider the following:

- **S**ite: The outer area of the knee.

- **T**ype: An aching pain, closer to the surface than the previous two ligaments. It might be a sharp pain when it first happens. The knee might also feel unstable, lock, or catch. It will often be tender to touch and there may be swelling on the outside of the knee. There will usually be a popping noise when it first happens.

- **O**nset: Sudden, usually because of a direct blow or force to the inside of the knee, which pushes the knee outwards and damages the LCL.

- **P**rovoked: Discomfort when walking, standing, putting pressure on the affected side.

MEDIAL COLLATERAL LIGAMENT (MCL)

The MCL ligament is the counterpart to the LCL. It is another long ligament that is close to the surface, but this time on the inside of the knee. It attaches the femur in the thigh to the thick shin bone called the tibia. Along with the LCL, it is responsible for the sideways stability of the knee and stops the knee joint from sliding too far inwards.

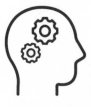

For MCL sprains or tears, start with your pain scale and **STOP** and then consider the following:

- **S**ite: The inside of the knee.

- **T**ype: It will usually be a sharp pain when it first happens, which reduces to a dull ache. There will normally be tenderness around the inside of the knee. It will feel unstable, as if your knee is going to give way. There may also be swelling and bruising. There will usually be a popping noise when it first happens.

- **O**nset: Sudden, usually because of a direct blow to the outside of the knee, which pushes the knee inwards and damages the MCL. It can also happen because of a repeated force moving the knee inwards or quick, sudden movements of the knee.

- **P**rovoked: Discomfort when walking, standing, putting pressure on the affected side.

SELF-HELP

- At home you should try **R**est, **I**ce, **C**ompression and **E**levation to help reduce the inflammation (see page 70). Gentle self-massage on the quad and hamstring muscles can also help.

- You should see a doctor, physiotherapist, chiropractor or osteopath to diagnose these conditions. The diagnosis will usually need to be confirmed by an MRI scan as the extent of the tear will need to be known for the ACL and PCL ligaments.

- A tear to the ACL or PCL ligaments is more serious than the other two surface ligaments. If someone came to me with a suspected tear of these two smaller, deeper ligaments, I would provide conservative treatment to try and help reduce the swelling, by using massage to try and drain fluid away from the knee. Cold laser therapy can also help with this process. I would then advise the client to have an urgent MRI scan.

- If there is a complete tear, or a severe partial tear, you will often need surgery if it is the PCL or ACL ligament. It's rare that you will have a complete rupture to the MCL or LCL, so it's more likely to be a partial tear, which you don't normally need surgery for.

- The main aim of treatment with an acute tear is to reduce the swelling, and Tecar therapy can help with this.

- Once the inflammation is gone, and if it's a partial tear, I try to work on the balance of the knee, massaging the tight muscles and using dry needling as well. Gentle mobilization can help, but this must be done carefully so that you don't stress the ligament even more.

- Once the healing is well under way, a therapist should then help you explore what has made these ligaments vulnerable and treat those areas as well. There might be an imbalance in the muscles of the knees or an issue with the quads, ankles, or hips.

THE UNHAPPY TRIAD

The 'unhappy triad', or 'blown knee', is when an impact injury or trauma is so bad that the ACL, MCL, and medial meniscus are all damaged (see Figure 13.4). It requires such force that it only usually happens in contact sports or car accidents. If surgery is needed, then it will normally only be needed for the ACL and medial meniscus, as the MCL can usually repair on its own. There is more about the medial meniscus in the following section.

FIG. 13.4
UNHAPPY TRIAD KNEE INJURY

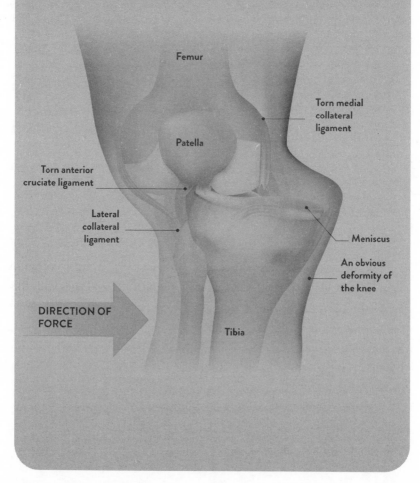

Femur

Torn medial
collateral
ligament

Patella

Torn anterior
cruciate ligament

Lateral
collateral
ligament

Meniscus

An obvious
deformity of
the knee

DIRECTION OF
FORCE

Tibia

CARTILAGE TEAR

Cartilage is a smooth elastic tissue that covers the ends of bones and insides of joints to stop them from rubbing against each other. If you had a bird's-eye view of the inside of the knee, you would see that the menisci are two crescent-shaped structures that face each other. They act as shock absorbers and cushions between the femur and tibia bones and help the bones move smoothly (see Figure 13.5).

FIG. 13.5
MENISCUS CARTILAGE

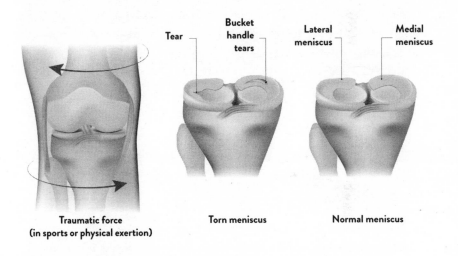

Traumatic force
(in sports or physical exertion)   **Torn meniscus**   **Normal meniscus**

The meniscus cartilage in the knee is one of the most common areas of cartilage to tear, and I regularly see clients of all ages with this injury. In younger people, it usually occurs when playing sport when the knee is twisted forcefully or rotated while also having most of the body's weight on it. I see a lot of netball players with this condition. I would even go so far as to say that there is an epidemic of meniscus tears, as well as ACL tears, among teenage netball players as they are not allowed to dribble the ball, so the players must turn and twist while keeping their feet firmly planted on the ground – all the right ingredients for a cartilage tear.

In older people, damage to the meniscus is usually due to wear and tear. There is a weakening of the cartilage and surrounding structures, until it's torn during a more minor twisting action such as stumbling when standing up from sitting. In older people there might not even be a memorable event that preceded it. Back in Chapter 2, I talked about my client, Sonia, who had been lying on her couch because of pain in her back. You might remember that the original pain that made her adjust her behaviour was from her knee. She had torn her meniscus after years of standing for work and noticed a low-level pain on the outside of her knee. One day at work, she made a normal twisting action to reach for something on a shelf and tore the cartilage in her knee.

Meniscus tears often happen because the quad is tight, and this puts too much force on the cartilage. It's therefore important to massage around the quads when treating a meniscal tear.

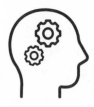 Start with your pain scale and **STOP**, and then consider the following:

- **S**ite: On either side of the knee.

- **T**ype: It can be a sharp or stabbing pain at first, ranging from mild to severe, which will then turn into a dull ache. There might be a locking sensation when moving the knee, and the knee will usually be swollen.

- **O**nset: It will be sudden, usually with a forceful twisting or rotating of the knee. The older you are the less dramatic the twisting action will need to be to tear the meniscus.

- **P**rovoked by: Straightening the knee, twisting or rotating the knee, squatting, or going up and down stairs.

It can be quite difficult to tell the difference between a potential ligament injury and a meniscus tear. With a ligament tear there is usually a loud popping noise, which doesn't normally happen with a meniscus. The only ligament that doesn't often make this noise is the PCL. Another clue for a ligament tear is that the knee will feel unstable and can't take your weight, whereas it won't feel so unstable with a meniscus tear.

SELF-HELP

- At home, you should try some self-massage on the quads, which are the thigh muscles above the knee.

PROFESSIONAL HELP

- You can see either a physiotherapist, chiropractor, or osteopath for this condition.

- First, it needs to be diagnosed, and there are a lot of orthopaedic tests that a therapist or doctor will use. It's best that these are carried out by either a therapist or doctor as they might cause more damage if it's actually a ligament tear and the tests aren't performed by someone who is appropriately qualified. A general test for a meniscus tear is trying to notice if there is more pain when your knee rotates or twists. If this happens, then it's likely to be a meniscus tear.

- When I see patients with meniscus tears, I normally start by asking the client to bend their knee. This allows me to position dry needles right inside the joint space down to the crescent where the meniscus is. I then massage the quad muscles and test the knee again to see if it is still locking or catching. I do this with all the muscles around the knee until I find the one that is the root cause of the issue.

- Laser therapy is very good for meniscus tears as it can go directly to the cartilage.

- The aim of any treatment should be to restore function without aggravating the meniscus further. Once it's beginning to heal, you can then gently try and strengthen the knee, but this must be done carefully so you don't re-injure yourself.

MYTH BUSTERS

Not all ligament and meniscus injuries need surgery to repair them. There are other options (outlined in the treatment section), particularly with incomplete tears. Before going down the surgery route, I would see a physiotherapist, chiropractor or osteopath who can help restore function to the tissue.

OSTEOARTHRITIS

Of all the areas of the body, osteoarthritis is most commonly seen in the knees. For more about arthritis take a look at Chapter 3 but, in brief, osteoarthritis occurs in the knee when the protective cartilage becomes damaged and wears away. The bones then begin to rub on each other causing pain and swelling. Knee replacement surgery isn't inevitable when it comes to osteoarthritis. There are plenty of other therapies than can help before surgery needs to be considered.

The patients I normally see with this kind of osteoarthritis are over the age of 45, runners, or people who have been doing manual jobs for years. It is also thought to be hereditary in some cases, and is more common in women than men. I have tried to avoid bringing people's weight into any of these sections, because I strongly believe that a healthy body isn't always a skinny one, but when it comes to osteoarthritis of the knee, most of the patients I see are overweight. There is a direct link between weight and this condition. Therefore, if you are overweight and have osteoarthritis in your knee, it will help ease the pressure on your knees if you do manage to lose some of those extra pounds.

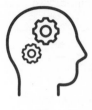

Start with your pain scale and **STOP**, and then consider the following:

- **S**ite: Around the knee.

- **T**ype: A dull ache. There can also be stiffness, swelling, a clicking or creaking sound, or a grinding sensation when moving the knee.

- **O**nset: Gradual.

- **P**rovoked: Activity generally makes it worse, including walking, going up stairs, and repetitive bending. It is often worse in the mornings.

SELF-HELP

- There is a fine line to tread with osteoarthritis of the knee as resting helps alleviate pain, which is always important. But not using the knee enough will gradually see the range of movement in the joint reduce. Therefore, try to remain active if you can, even if you feel like retreating to the couch.

- You can see either a physiotherapist, chiropractor, or osteopath for this condition.

- The therapist's aim should be to regain the lost movement in the knee by gently massaging the muscles surrounding it.

- The treatment that works best on osteoarthritis of the knee is cold laser therapy. I recommend it to all my clients who have this condition.

OTHER COMMON KNEE CONDITIONS

- The *iliotibial band* (IT band) is a long thick tendon that runs down the outside of the thigh and connects the tensor fasciae latae (TFL) muscle to the knee joint (see also Chapter 12). The IT band's job is to stabilize the knee joint and it can become strained, which can cause referred pain to the knee or hip. It is most commonly strained in runners through overuse. However, because it's a tendon, it's supposed to feel tight and is often over massaged when there is nothing wrong with it. If you suspect a problem with your IT band, before pummelling it with a foam roller every day, it's best to go to an experienced therapist who will help diagnose the condition.

- *Bursitis* is inflammation of one of the four bursae in the knee. There is more about bursitis in Chapter 3. The most common bursa in the knee to become inflamed is the prepatellar, which is above the kneecap.

- *Osgood Schlatter's* is a disease that causes pain and swelling in the tibia bone below the kneecap. It's most common in children between ages 9 and 14 who play a lot of sport, as it's linked to overuse while going through a growth spurt.

- *Baker's cyst* is a cyst that forms at the back of the knee due to inflammation of the tissue there. It can cause locking or a catching sensation in the knee. The cyst can sometimes burst and leak down into the calf, which will cause pain, redness, and swelling in the calf.

STRETCHES AND EXERCISES FOR THE KNEE

With knee conditions, we must be careful not to stress our knees while we are still healing. I've therefore only included a couple of gentle exercises for this section which can be increased as your recovery progresses. As with all the exercises in the book, if they are painful or make your injury worse, then please stop them immediately.

FIG. 13.6
SELF-MASSAGE TECHNIQUES FOR THE KNEE

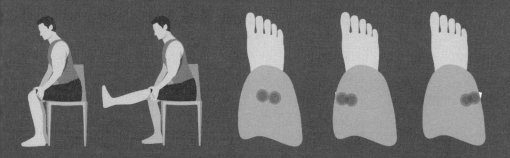

1

My favourite self-massage technique is for the quads, as they are often the root cause of most knee injuries. Sit with your feet on the floor and place both hands on one knee above the joint. Wrap your finger pads around the back of your knee, leaving your thumbs at the front of your leg. Firmly grip the area above the kneecap with your thumbs and bend and straighten your knee ten times. Move your thumbs to the other positions in Figure 13.6 and bend and straighten the knee ten times for each one. Repeat all of this on the other knee.

2

Small squats, when you are only bending the knee slightly, are a good place to start when introducing exercise to a healed knee. Place your hands on your hips and move your legs shoulder-width apart. Bend both your legs to only twenty or thirty degrees. Even this small amount of movement will help to lubricate the joint. When you feel that your knee is healed, you can increase the depth of the squats to help strengthen the knee.

CHAPTER 14

Foot
and ankle

T he thing I always notice with feet is that they come in all shapes and sizes, and often their owners wish they were different. Some people have one foot larger than the other, some have flat feet, and others have high arches, but all of them usually perform their primary job of supporting our entire weight while allowing us to balance, walk, run, and jump.

Each of your feet has twenty-eight bones (including the sesamoid bones). This means that 27 per cent of your bones are in both of your feet. There are also thirty-three joints and over 100 muscles, tendons, and ligaments – it's a very busy area.

The feet also act as shock absorbers and both the heels and arches help with this. High arches or flat feet can sometimes cause problems with our joints and the muscles higher up, so it's always good to be aware if you have one of the following conditions (see Figure 14.1).

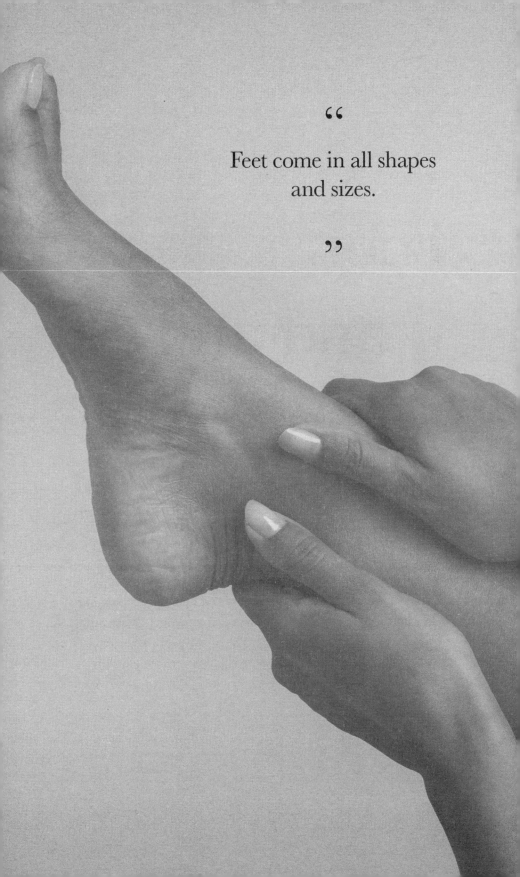

"

Feet come in all shapes
and sizes.

"

FIG. 14.1
DEFORMATION OF THE FOOT

FLAT FEET

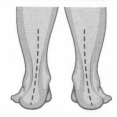 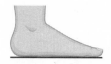 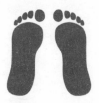

Your foot rolls inwards when you walk

Your body weight goes towards the inner foot

The inner arch is flattened or decreased

Poor absorption of body weight can affect muscles and joints in the knee, hip, leg, and lower back

You can alleviate this condition with footwear that supports your arch

NEUTRAL

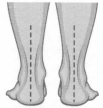 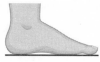 

The foot doesn't roll inwards or outwards

Your arch will naturally support your body weight

HIGH ARCH

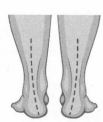 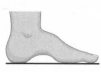 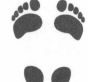

Your foot rolls outwards when you walk

Your body weight goes towards the outer foot

This can lead to bone, tendon, and ligament problems around the outer foot and ankle, as well as muscle and joint issues higher up in the body

You can see a podiatrist if you suspect you have a high arch

ARE YOUR FEET AND ANKLES HEALTHY?

Healthy feet and ankles should be able to do the following without any pain:

1
Move your toes up and down (this is called an *active* movement)

2
Place your index finger and thumb on either side of your big toe and move it up and down, and from side to side (this is called a *passive* movement)

3
Move your ankle clockwise and anticlockwise

4
Stand on your tiptoes

5
Place your body weight on both heels

Even though we should be aware of our flat feet or high arches, people with these conditions are still capable of reaching the highest level of sporting achievements. Like a lot of Black people, I have flat feet. I've also seen flat feet and raised arches on some of our greatest sportspeople. Therefore, although we should be aware of the conditions and try to alleviate any symptoms they may produce, we shouldn't necessarily believe that they will hold us back.

As an osteopath, I can honestly say that feet are one of my favourite areas of the body to treat. They often help me identify problems in the joints and muscles higher up in the body and are also very responsive to treatment. Flat feet and raised arches can come alive again through mobilization of the joints that form the arches, and this in itself can rejuvenate the feet.

THE BEST TIME FOR SHOE SHOPPING
The wrong footwear and incorrect size of shoe can cause many problems in the feet. You should therefore buy your shoes at the end of the working day, as your feet are more swollen then and slightly larger.

There are three arches in the foot, rather than one, and these are all made from joints (see Figure 14.2).

FIG. 14.2
THE ARCHES OF THE FOOT

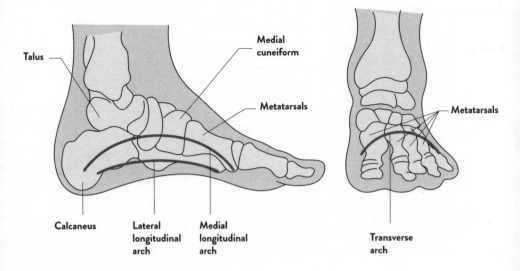

Talus

Medial cuneiform

Metatarsals

Metatarsals

Calcaneus

Lateral longitudinal arch

Medial longitudinal arch

Transverse arch

The ankle is a hinge joint that connects the fibula and tibia bones in the lower leg to the talus bone, which is the first bone in the foot and the keystone of the ankle (see Figure 14.3). There are two joints in the ankle. The true ankle joint allows the up and down motion, while the subtalar joint enables the side-to-side movements of the foot. If the ankle has lost its mobility or is even slightly out of sync it can have repercussions on the rest of the body, all the way up to the lower back, including the sacroiliac (SI) joints. It's therefore important that we are all aware of any potential problems in the ankle. The best place to start is by going through the above tests for your foot and ankle health, at the start of the chapter.

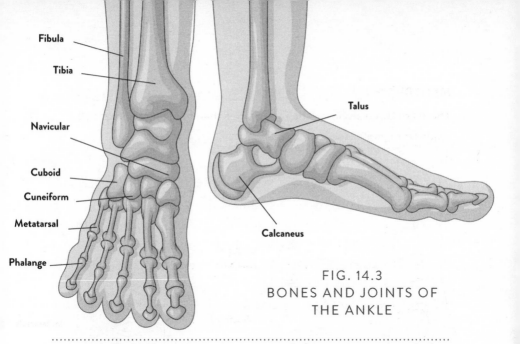

FIG. 14.3
BONES AND JOINTS OF
THE ANKLE

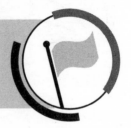

There are several warning flags when it comes to the foot and ankle, so always seek urgent medical attention if you experience any of the following:

- Not being able to weight-bear

- The pain is worse at night

- Joints are hot

- Trauma

- History of osteoporosis

- Extreme swelling that isn't alleviated by anything

- Swelling for no apparent reason

- History of cancer

- Unexplained weight loss

- Weakness in the foot or both feet

- Pins and needles or numbness in both feet

- A suspected fracture to the foot

MOST COMMON FOOT AND ANKLE CONDITIONS: PLANTAR FASCIITIS

The plantar fascia is a connective tissue at the bottom of the foot that links the heel bone to the toes. It helps support one arch and acts as a shock absorber. Plantar fasciitis is a common condition that happens when this tissue becomes inflamed after being overworked (see Figure 14.4).

This is an incredibly common condition among people aged 40 to 60, and the clients I see with it often walk or stand for long periods throughout the day. Being overweight, having tight calf muscles, and ill-fitting footwear can all be contributing factors. High arches or flat feet can also lead to plantar fasciitis, but it often happens to people with a neutral arch as well.

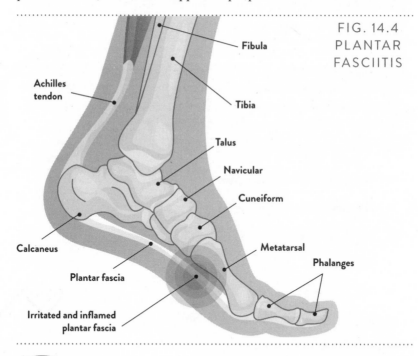

FIG. 14.4
PLANTAR
FASCIITIS

Fibula

Achilles
tendon

Tibia

Talus

Navicular

Cuneiform

Calcaneus

Metatarsal

Phalanges

Plantar fascia

Irritated and inflamed
plantar fascia

Start with your pain scale and **STOP**, and then consider the following:

- **S**ite: Sole of the foot, near the heel bone. It usually occurs in one foot rather than both at the same time.

- **T**ype: It can be a dull ache or stabbing/sharp pain, depending on your activities during the day. It can often be too tender to touch.

- **O**nset: It will be a gradual onset.

- **P**rovoked: It is often worse in the mornings, when standing for long periods, getting up from sitting, and weight-bearing. It can often be worse following exercise rather than during it.

PATIENT FILES: PLANTAR FASCIITIS

Monica had been feeling pain in the sole of her foot for almost two weeks when she came to visit me. She'd felt a sharp pain every morning with her first couple of steps. Having never had any problems with her feet before, she couldn't understand where the pain had come from. I examined her feet and it was clearly plantar fasciitis that had been caused by a tight heel arch and lack of movement in her big toe, which had put additional strain on the plantar fascia and aggravated it. Her heel was very tender so I first used cold laser therapy, which then enabled me to lightly massage the muscles around the heel. I then restored the movement to the tight muscles in her big toe and heel arch through massage, which took the pressure away from the plantar fascia.

SELF-HELP

- If you can't rest your heel, you can buy gel pads from a chemist to put into your shoe that can reduce the pain temporarily. Even part of a sponge can be cut up and placed in your shoe and this should help take the pressure off your heel.

- If it is a chronic condition and you are overweight, losing some of those extra pounds can take the pressure off the plantar fascia.

- **R**est, **I**ce, **C**ompression, and **E**levation can help alleviate any swelling and inflammation (see page 70).

- At home, running a golf ball or tennis ball along the sole of the foot and away from the tender area can help loosen the muscles (see Figure 14.5).

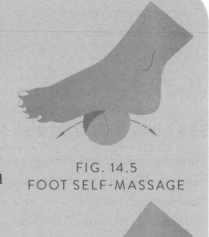

FIG. 14.5
FOOT SELF-MASSAGE

PROFESSIONAL HELP

- You can see an osteopath, chiropractor or physiotherapist for treatment. If the therapist suspects that there are problems with your arches, then it may be useful to have this checked by a podiatrist.

- A therapist can help with mobilization of the feet and taking the pressure off the arch and plantar fascia. I massage the leg muscles as there are several tendons that reach into the foot. If they are tense, then they can aggravate the plantar fascia. I then use massage and mobilization on the joints in the arches and massage the small muscles in the feet. Depending on how tender the plantar fascia is, I either massage it or use dry needling.

- The heel of the foot is the most sensitive area of the body to dry needle and isn't always pain-free, but my clients have reported that the area is less sensitive afterwards.

- If the area is very tender to touch, I use cold laser therapy or Tecar therapy.

SPRAINS AND TEARS TO ANKLE LIGAMENTS

There are several large ligaments around the ankle, which help to stabilize it and prevent excessive movements (see Figure 14.6). These ligaments are damaged when the ankle is forced beyond its normal range of movement. The rolling or twisting of the ankle, or a rapid change in direction, or awkward movement can all cause a sprain or tear to these ligaments.

The clients I normally see with ligament damage are aged between 30 and 40 and are usually male. The most common ligaments to tear are the ones on the outside of the ankle as often our ankles buckle and roll outwards (see Figure 14.7).

The following text only deals with the outer ligaments of the ankle, as these are far more easily damaged than the inner ones. There is more information about ligaments in Chapter 3.

PATIENT FILES: LIGAMENT STRAIN

Gabriela was going down the stairs when she tripped and twisted her ankle. She was unable to weight-bear afterwards so went to A&E where she was diagnosed with a ligament sprain. She visited me a couple of days later for treatment. I used electroacupuncture to help reduce the pain and this allowed me to massage the area to encourage drainage and reduce the swelling. The following week, I used mobilization to aid movement in the ankle. A week after that, Gabriela was able to weight-bear fully.

FIG. 14.6
LIGAMENTS IN THE ANKLE JOINT

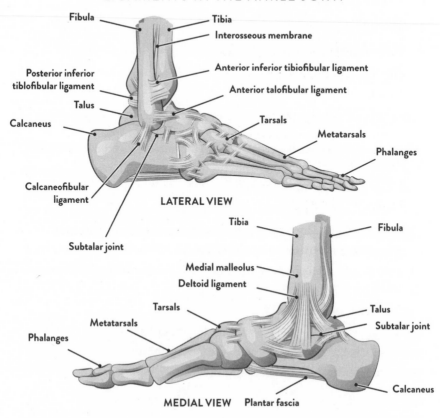

Fibula

Tibia

Interosseous membrane

Anterior inferior tibiofibular ligament

Posterior inferior tiblofibular ligament

Anterior talofibular ligament

Talus

Calcaneus

Tarsals

Metatarsals

Phalanges

Calcaneofibular ligament

LATERAL VIEW

Subtalar joint

Tibia

Fibula

Medial malleolus

Deltoid ligament

Talus

Tarsals

Subtalar joint

Metatarsals

Phalanges

Calcaneus

MEDIAL VIEW   Plantar fascia

FIG. 14.7
TYPES OF ANKLE SPRAINS

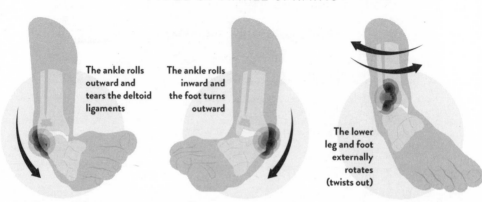

The ankle rolls outward and tears the deltoid ligaments

The ankle rolls inward and the foot turns outward

The lower leg and foot externally rotates (twists out)

INVERSION ANKLE SPRAINS

EVERSION ANKLE SPRAINS

HIGH ANKLE SPRAINS

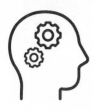

Start with your pain scale and **STOP**, and then consider the following:

- **S**ite: Outer part of the ankle.

- **T**ype: It will be a sharp pain when first done, then a dull ache with a sharper pain on movement. There will be a lot of swelling if it's torn and some swelling with a sprain, depending on the severity. It will often be bruised and tender to touch. There may be a popping sensation or sound.

- **O**nset: It can be sudden, normally following a fall, twisting movement, or blow to the ankle. If it's a sprain, rather than a tear, it can either be gradual or sudden.

- **P**rovoked by: Rolling your foot outwards, weight-bearing, and general movements of the ankle.

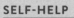

SELF-HELP

- You shouldn't take anti-inflammatory medication, such as Ibuprofen, in the first forty-eight hours as the initial inflammation aids the healing of the ligament.

- **R**est, **I**ce, **C**ompression, and **E**levation can help alleviate any swelling (see page 70).

- Once a tear is healed, then restoring the range of movement is important. Take a look at the exercises at the bottom of the chapter for more information on this. If you can afford it, it's a good idea to see a physiotherapist as they will help strengthen the ankle and prevent further injuries. If you've twisted an ankle in the past, then it can make you prone to damaging the ligaments again.

- You can see a physiotherapist, chiropractor or osteopath for this condition. You might need to see a doctor or have an MRI scan if there is a severe or complete tear.

- Treatment will vary depending on whether it is a sprain or tear. If it's a sprain, then the therapist will be able to work directly on the site of the sprain and use massage to ease the tension in the ligament and surrounding muscles. If there is a tear, it's better to work remotely on the muscles around the ankle or use non-invasive treatments. If the area is tender to touch, I use Tecar therapy. Cold laser therapy also helps with swelling and pain relief.

- Electroacupuncture is very beneficial for healing damaged ligaments.

ACHILLES TENDON

The Achilles tendon is a large tendon at the back of the ankle that links the heel to two of the calf muscles (see Figure 14.8). This tendon is very important as it enables us to flex and extend our feet, and is intrinsic in allowing us to walk and run. The Achilles tendon is also the largest tendon in the body.

It's very common to damage the Achilles tendon, and this can be a simple sprain all the way through to a complete tear. In my experience, a complete tear is mostly seen among men aged between 30 and 40. Clients have described it as though they have been kicked in the back of the leg and there is usually an audible popping noise.

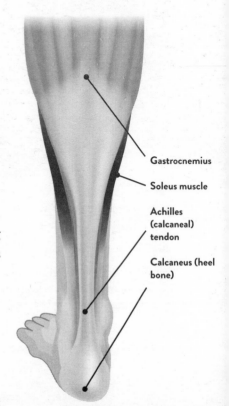

FIG. 14.8
ACHILLES TENDON
AND CALF MUSCLES

Gastrocnemius

Soleus muscle

Achilles (calcaneal) tendon

Calcaneus (heel bone)

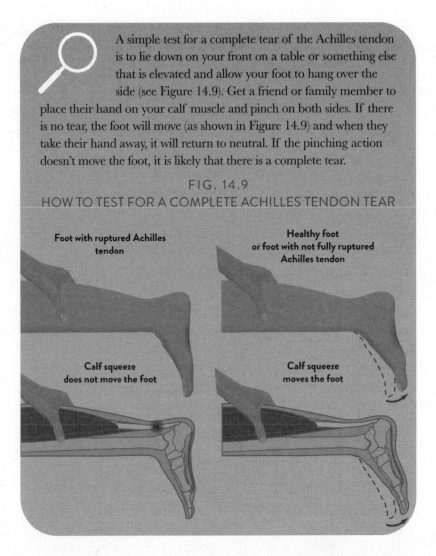

A simple test for a complete tear of the Achilles tendon is to lie down on your front on a table or something else that is elevated and allow your foot to hang over the side (see Figure 14.9). Get a friend or family member to place their hand on your calf muscle and pinch on both sides. If there is no tear, the foot will move (as shown in Figure 14.9) and when they take their hand away, it will return to neutral. If the pinching action doesn't move the foot, it is likely that there is a complete tear.

FIG. 14.9
HOW TO TEST FOR A COMPLETE ACHILLES TENDON TEAR

Foot with ruptured Achilles tendon

Healthy foot or foot with not fully ruptured Achilles tendon

Calf squeeze does not move the foot

Calf squeeze moves the foot

When it comes to lesser injuries or conditions of the Achilles tendons, they are either strains, minor tears, or inflammation. The people I see most with these conditions are runners, or people who have been inactive for a long time before taking up sport, or clients who haven't allowed themselves enough rest time between workout sessions.

Both strains and inflammation of the Achilles tendon have similar symptoms and treatment requirements, so I will deal with them as one below. The following advice isn't for ruptures of the Achilles tendon as they are relatively rare.

PATIENT FILES: ACHILLES TENDON STRAIN

Emily was a keen runner and had even joined a local running club. She would feel a low-level pain in both her Achilles tendons at around a two or three on the pain scale after running. She was also stiff around her calves in the morning. She had changed her running shoes multiple times, but nothing had helped. Over the months, the pain gradually grew worse until it was a six on the pain scale after running. This is when she came to see me. I worked on loosening up her calf muscles and mobilizing her feet. What helped her the most was doing ankle exercises every day. I also analysed her running technique, and it was clear that this was also putting pressure on her Achilles tendon. A few small changes, and she was able to enjoy running again.

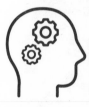 For strains, inflammation, and minor tears of the Achilles tendon, start with your pain scale and **STOP** and then consider the following:

- **S**ite: Can be in one specific part of the Achilles tendon, such as the heel or mid-calf, or it can spread throughout the whole tendon.

- **T**ype: Can be the full range from a mild to sharp pain. There will be stiffness in the lower leg, particularly in the morning or after resting. It can be tender to touch. There might be lumps, nodules, or a thickening of the tendon.

- **O**nset: It can either be sudden or gradual. With a gradual onset, there will be hints of pain that often disappear for a time.

- **P**rovoked by: Going up stairs, running, wearing high heels, and raising the lower leg.

FIG. 14.10
STRENGTHENING EXERCISE FOR ACHILLES TENDON

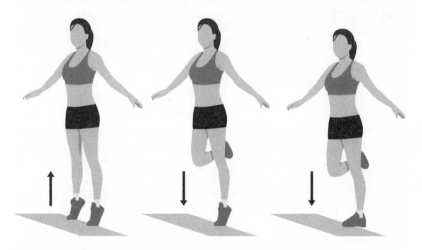

PROFESSIONAL HELP

- You can see a physiotherapist, chiropractor or osteopath for these conditions.

- In most cases, problems with the Achilles tendon happen because there is an imbalance in the calf muscles, so I would start with massaging them to loosen any tightness. The joints in the foot and ankle will also need to be loosened through mobilization as they are often tight. The plantar fascia should also be massaged – the Achilles tendon really does need global treatment.

- If the Achilles tendon isn't too tender to touch, I start by massaging all of it. The sides are just as important as the middle and often get ignored. If the tendon is too tender to touch, I dry needle the areas around it first.

- A gait analysis can be useful as this will often show what is irritating the tendon.

OTHER COMMON FOOT AND ANKLE CONDITIONS

- *Gout* is a type of arthritis that most commonly affects the big toe, but can affect other joints. The onset will often be sudden and the pain severe. The big toe can feel warm and appear red. It is more common in men than women, but menopausal women can be prone to it. It will be diagnosed through a blood test and scan.

- *Bunions* are very common among women who wear high heels, but bunions can also be caused by pointy shoes, ill-fitting shoes, and arthritis, and can even be hereditary. Bunions occur when the bones in the feet shift out of sync (see Figure 14.11) and can only be restored with surgery.

FIG. 14.11
MOVEMENT OF BONE WITH BUNIONS

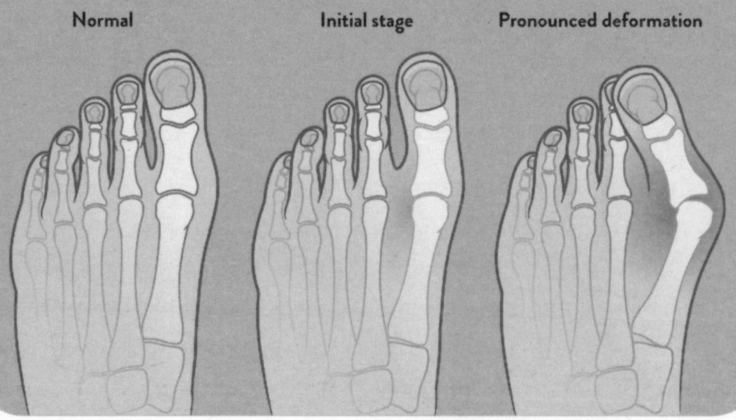

Normal   Initial stage   Pronounced deformation

- Underneath your big toe are two sesamoid bones (see Figure 14.12), and if these become irritated and inflamed it's called *sesamoiditis*. These bones act as shock absorbers, and symptoms of sesamoiditis are swelling and redness around the big toe. It will also be difficult to move the big toe up and down. Surgery is commonly offered for this condition but loosening up the flexor hallucis longus (FHL) muscle in the back of the calf, as well as the muscles on the sole of the foot, can often help alleviate the pressure and give the sesamoid bones a chance to heal.

FIG. 14.12
SESAMOID BONES IN THE FOOT

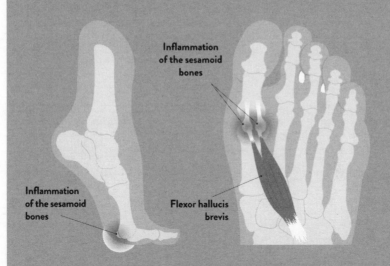

Inflammation of the sesamoid bones

Inflammation of the sesamoid bones

Flexor hallucis brevis

- I have seen several patients who suffer from numbness in their feet because they have *diabetes*. Not being able to feel sensations in any area of the body can be dangerous so you should see your doctor about this.

- A *foot drop* is when you cannot move your foot upwards and is discussed in more detail in Chapter 2. The most common cause of a foot drop is a disc herniation pressing on the L5 nerve in the lower back.

STRETCHES AND EXERCISES FOR THE FOOT AND ANKLE

There are so many useful stretches and exercises for the feet and ankles, and I have chosen a selection that will be beneficial at each stage of your recovery. As with all the exercises in the book, if they are painful or make your injury worse then please stop them immediately.

FIG. 14.13
SELF-MASSAGE FOR THE FEET

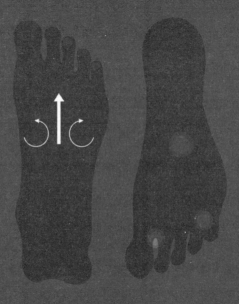

1

Self-massage is great for the feet. You can use circular motions over the top of your feet and massage between the bones and toes. You can do this with oil or with dry hands. You can also press on the sole of your feet to find trigger points (as shown in Figure 14.13) and press and hold these for five seconds.

2

If you have an injured foot or ankle and have been told not to weight-bear, or if weight-bearing hurts too much, you can keep them mobile, while staying seated, by trying to write the alphabet in capital letters with your foot.

FIG. 14.14

STRENGTHENING EXERCISES FOR FOOT AND ANKLE USING A RESISTANCE BAND

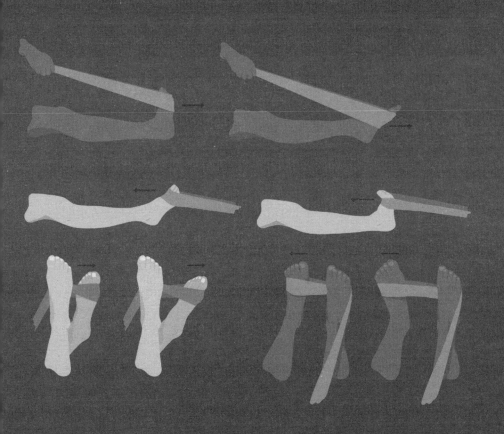

3

A resistance band is cheap to buy and useful for strengthening the foot and ankle. Try the different moves shown in Figure 14.14. Each one should be done ten times a day. You may want to ask a friend to hold the band, or tie it around a stable object for some of these.

4

When you have recovered, you can try some weight-bearing exercises. A simple one is, when standing, to raise yourself on to your tiptoes and then gently bring your heels down. Do this ten times. You can also do this on one leg and hold for five seconds, gradually building up to ten seconds.

PART THREE:

Therapists and Therapies

CHAPTER 15

Working with
a therapist

A therapist is someone who specializes in a particular treatment (or several treatments) that will help you feel better. You might have an idea of what your diagnosis might be, but which type of therapist do you choose? And how do you pick the best therapist in your local area?

If I had to choose a new therapist, I would start by finding out what each one has in their toolbox. There are some grey areas between specialisms as some skills overlap and, most importantly, the therapist might have had additional training in other treatments. Check their website to see what they offer. Do they do dry needling? Are they experienced with clicking and mobilization? Do they provide any other treatments? And, most importantly, are they prepared to use them all in a single session rather than having a session for clicking, a session for massage, a session for dry needling, and so on. Most therapies can be combined in a single session and, wherever possible, they should be.

A therapist might also have a specialism. Some might excel in treating patients with hypermobility, others in sports injuries. That's not to say that they won't be perfectly competent in dealing with other conditions, but if you do have chronic fatigue and you can find someone who specializes in it then this will give you a head start when it comes to treatment.

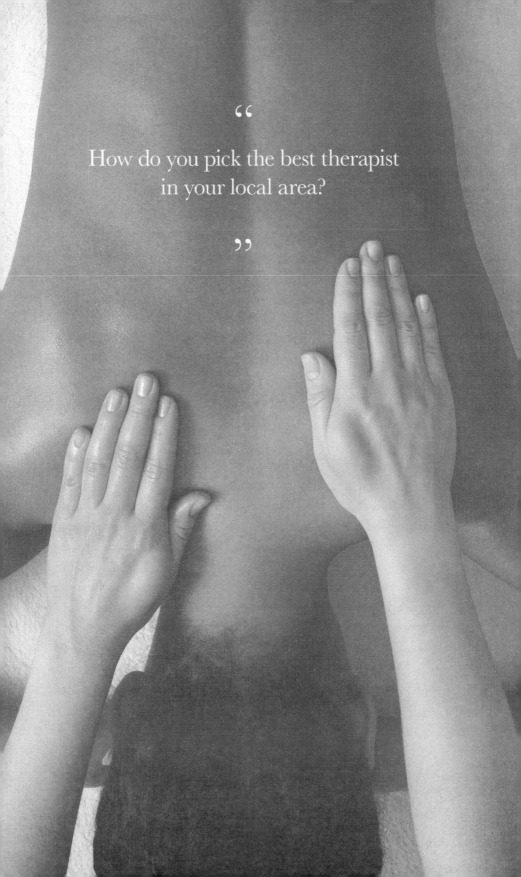

"

How do you pick the best therapist
in your local area?

"

It's all about getting the maximum benefit from the appointment. You are the client and will be paying a fee for their services if it's outside of the National Health Service (NHS), which provides free healthcare to anyone living in the United Kingdom. It's therefore best to come prepared. At your first session you will be asked a series of questions, called a 'case history', about your current health and past conditions and this reduces the time for treatment. If you are taking any medications, bring a list of them with you rather than rummaging through your bag or calling your doctor. Before the appointment, think about how you can clearly explain what the problem is and use your pain scale and STOP to guide you. Use the language of a therapist – if you suspect you might have overworked your upper trapezius muscles, say so. The therapist will know you are someone who has thought about their condition and researched it. The more relevant information they have, the quicker they can turn their mind to diagnosis and treatment. If it turns out it isn't your traps but is in fact your levator scapulae that is strained, they won't hold it against you as you were trying to point them in the right direction. You should expect some treatment during your first appointment, even if it's only ten minutes, so don't let a lengthy form take that away from you.

> ## "EXPLAIN WHAT THE PROBLEM IS AND USE YOUR PAIN SCALE AND STOP TO GUIDE YOU."

TIP

When seeing a doctor or therapist, remember your pain scale and **STOP**. These will provide a strong, succinct grounding for explaining your condition.

Take this approach with your doctor as well. Time is precious with those appointments too. Practise how you are going to explain your pain by running through your pain scale and STOP. All this information supplies the clues for them to eventually arrive at a diagnosis. General practitioners are the gateway to accessing specialists in the NHS, so any relevant information you can provide is always beneficial.

When choosing a therapist, always start with a recommendation from a family member or friend if you can. When I was in full-time private practice, I received most of my work by word of mouth and recommendations.

"A GOOD THERAPIST WILL MAKE YOU FEEL LIKE AN INDIVIDUAL NOT JUST ANOTHER NUMBER."

When you are being treated, it's key that the therapist doesn't just concentrate on the area where you are feeling pain. If you have a problem with your shoulder and don't receive any treatment for your neck and back, then it might be time to find a new therapist. A good therapist will make you feel like an individual, not just another number coming through the door that they are rushing to process. A great therapist will do all of this and when you leave the session you will also have:

- An idea of what the problem is, or a route to diagnosis.

- Alleviated some of your pain

- A plan in place for how you will tackle the condition both from therapy and at home

If you don't think that any of these three things have been addressed, or there isn't a good reason why they haven't, it might be time to find a new therapist.

The therapist should also be able to convey this information to you in a language you understand; if they don't, ask for an explanation. It might be that you are someone who learns better through visual explanations, rather than verbal ones, so they should be happy to explain your condition with a diagram or model if this is the case. It is their job to translate medical language into something you can easily understand and in an empathetic way. If they refuse or are unable to do that, ask yourself why. It might be that they're not sure of what's going on themselves, and are trying to hide this behind the complexity and formality of their words.

Finally, it's all about honesty. Not everyone will know straightaway what's wrong with you, and I count myself in this group as well. If a therapist doesn't know what's wrong, they should tell you. If they aren't the right specialist, they should tell you. It doesn't lessen their abilities and there shouldn't be any egos involved when it comes to a patient's health. The therapist should then refer the client on, or explain what the next steps for diagnosis are. There are different ways to get from A to Z: a therapist might have their own system of dry needling, or might use a different treatment that others don't have access to. The important thing is that you get to Z, and if a therapist can't do this—which happens to all of us—then they should tell you so, explain why, and refer you to another specialist or doctor. To help you with this, we'll now run through the main types of therapists you could see in the UK.

OSTEOPATHS

Osteopaths believe in treating the body as a whole and therefore the skeleton, muscles, ligaments, and connective tissues must work well together. One of their guiding principles is that each part of your body has a particular role, and if an area is damaged or injured then your body as a whole cannot function in the way it was intended. Another guiding principle, therefore, is osteopaths believe that 'structure governs function and function governs structure'. Osteopaths train for four years so that they are able to diagnose wide-ranging conditions. They treat the body's structures through massage, mobilization, and manipulation (clicking) of the joints, as well as encouraging the circulation of blood throughout the body to all the tissues.

Osteopathy was founded in the late nineteenth century in America by Andrew Taylor Still, who was a physician and surgeon. One of his students brought this new practice to the UK in 1913. Osteopathy is recognized by the World Health Organization (WHO), which published its own guidance on training in osteopathy in 2010.

Before starting treatment with an osteopath, you should check online with the General Osteopathic Council (osteopathy.org.uk) and see if your therapist is registered with them. This is a legal requirement for all osteopaths, and it is illegal to present yourself as a qualified osteopath if you are not registered with this organization.

An average session will last thirty to forty minutes, and you should receive some treatment even during a first session, if it is safe to do so. A therapist's prices will usually be shown on their website and you may have to pay more for the initial consultation.

In the session you should wear comfortable, loose clothing. For some therapists, and depending on the condition they are treating, you might not need to remove your clothing, whereas at other times you might be asked to remove your top and/or trousers. Osteopaths don't tend to use oil when they are massaging, but I always do. A good osteopath should not only treat the area where the client is feeling pain or discomfort. If the patient has a knee problem, then the ankles, hips, and lower back should also be checked. It's not as simple as 'the pain and therefore the root cause is confined to the knee' – everything is interlinked.

CHIROPRACTORS

Chiropractors specialize in the nervous system and focus on the diagnosis and treatment of disorders involving the muscles and nerves. They are known for treating neck and back conditions, but can cover all areas of the body. Their treatment predominantly involves mobilization or manipulation (clicking) of the joints and massage. They train for four years and believe that problems with the bones, muscles, and other tissues can affect the nervous system, and therefore

QUALIFIED

a patient's general health. Chiropractors often use X-rays to assist with a diagnosis and these will usually be taken by them in their clinic.

Chiropractic treatment was founded by Daniel David Palmer in America. It began in the late nineteenth century, around ten years after osteopathy first began. The name 'chiropractor' comes from the Greek language and means 'done by hand'. The British Chiropractic Society was established in 1925.

Before starting treatment with a chiropractor, you should check online with the General Chiropractic Council (www.gcc-uk.org) to see if your therapist is registered with them. This is a legal requirement for all chiropractors.

Appointments will usually be thirty minutes or less, although initial sessions will usually be longer. You can check a therapist's website for the cost of the appointment. Often an initial appointment will focus on an examination and diagnosis, and you will have to pay more for X-rays if they are needed. The diagnosis will often be presented to you in a report that you receive at the following appointment and a treatment plan will be outlined. The cost of the report will normally be included in the initial assessment fee. Some chiropractic clinics offer a subscription service where you are treated on a weekly or monthly basis. Chiropractors don't usually give out exercise plans, but this depends on the therapist, their specialisms, and postgraduate courses.

During an initial examination you may have to remove items of your clothing. Usually during a treatment session you won't have to remove any clothing unless you have a bulky jumper on, but it can depend on the therapist. Quite often chiropractic clinics have a specialist massage therapist who you will combine your treatment with.

> "THE NAME 'CHIROPRACTOR' COMES FROM THE GREEK LANGUAGE AND MEANS 'DONE BY HAND'."

PHYSIOTHERAPISTS

Physiotherapy takes a 'whole-person' approach to a patient and aims to restore function and movement to the body through exercises, massaging the tissues, and mobilization and manipulation of the joints. Patients are often provided with exercises to continue at home. Physiotherapy is widely used in the NHS and there are many specialisms within this setting including brain injuries, respiratory conditions, orthopaedics, and spinal-cord injuries.

In private practice, physiotherapists tend to concentrate more on rehabilitation following injuries or surgery, or work alongside sportspeople. They are trained to design exercise routines for weaknesses in a joint or muscle. Physios excel at rehabilitation plans and you should usually try and see one if you are in the recovery stage following a debilitating injury or surgery.

Physiotherapy has its core roots in the belief that exercise helps the body to remain healthy. On this basis, physiotherapy has been around for thousands of years. It has its formal roots in Sweden in the early nineteenth century with the introduction of the 'Swedish Movement' exercises, and in 1894, four nurses in the UK formed the Chartered Group of Physiotherapists.

> "PHYSIOS EXCEL AT REHABILITATION PLANS – TRY AND SEE ONE IF YOU ARE IN RECOVERY."

Unlike osteopathy or chiropractic treatment, physiotherapy is widely available on the NHS, so your doctor should be able to refer you to one. However, because of lengthy waiting lists, many people use a physiotherapist in private practice. If you take this route, you should check that they are qualified and registered with a recognized body such as the Chartered Society of Physiotherapists (www.csp.org.uk) and that they are also registered with the Health and Care Professions Council (hcpc-uk.org).

Physios are generally very good at orthopaedic testing as they normally work in the NHS first, where they see a variety of conditions compared to private practice. Osteopaths and chiropractors learn about all these conditions, but usually won't have dealt with as broad a range as physios. That said, osteopaths and chiropractors usually have more experience in dealing with injuries in the acute stage, whereas physios are more likely to work on the exercises for rehabilitation.

Physiotherapist appointments normally last between thirty and sixty minutes and details of their cost will usually be on the physiotherapist's website. Physiotherapy appointments may involve exercises or stretches, so try to wear comfortable clothing and trainers if you can.

MASSAGE THERAPIST

Massage therapists specialize in different massaging techniques or philosophies. Many different types of massage are available, spanning from Eastern philosophies through to sports therapies. I believe that the best therapists combine techniques during a session depending on the client's requirements, and they do this instinctively rather than expecting the client to choose what they have.

Elite sports teams and institutions have specialist massage therapists who only perform massage. If you can find someone who is an expert in this field they can help with your recovery, as well as keeping your body supple. In my opinion, massage is highly beneficial for preventing injuries, and there is more about massage therapy in Chapter 16.

"ELITE SPORTS TEAMS AND INSTITUTIONS HAVE SPECIALIST MASSAGE THERAPISTS."

Massage therapists don't generally have the medical training that osteopaths, chiropractors, and physiotherapists have. For this reason, I wouldn't recommend having treatment such as dry needling or clicking from a massage therapist, as they don't have the same background in surface anatomy, and it's difficult to find out how thorough their training in these other therapies has been.

Unlike physiotherapists, osteopaths, and chiropractors, there isn't a requirement for formal training for massage therapists, or a requirement for registration with a national organization before someone can set up their business. However, there are voluntary organizations such as the Complementary and Natural Healthcare Council (www.cnhc.org.uk) and the Federation of Holistic Therapists (www.fht.org.uk). If a therapist is registered with either one of these, it means that they have met their membership requirements. If I didn't have a recommendation from a family member or friend, I would start by searching these databases.

> "THERE ISN'T A REQUIREMENT FOR FORMAL TRAINING FOR MASSAGE THERAPISTS."

Sessions will normally last between thirty and sixty minutes. Be prepared to take most of your clothing off apart from your underwear. The therapist will normally drape towels over you to cover up the parts of your body that they are not working on.

PODIATRIST

Podiatry is a branch of medicine that deals with conditions and disorders of the feet and ankles. Another word for a podiatrist is a 'chiropodist' – podiatrist is the more modern term. Podiatrists can perform surgery on ingrown toenails, as well as deal with common conditions such as verrucas, corns, and fungal infections, as well as feet affected by diabetes. I mostly refer patients to podiatrists for heel-arch assessments, gait and running analysis or orthotics, as they are the experts in these areas. Podiatrists study for three years before qualifying.

Physicians have been caring for feet since the time of the Egyptians, but podiatry was always considered separate to conventional medicine of the time. This all changed when the first society of chiropodists was founded in America in the late nineteenth century. A similar society was set up in the UK in 1912.

You might be able to access podiatry through the NHS and you can speak to your doctor about this. However, most people will see a podiatrist on a private basis. If you take this route, you should check that they are registered with the Health and Care Professions Council (www.hcpc-uk.org). There are also several member organizations that they can register with as well, such as the British Chiropody and Podiatry Association (bcha-uk.org), which is always a good place to start when finding a podiatrist.

Appointments last from thirty to sixty minutes and their cost will usually be on the therapist's website. Complex matters such as surgery for an ingrown toenail or orthotics will incur an additional fee. A podiatrist will obviously want access to your feet during an appointment, but may also want to inspect further up your calf, so it's a good idea to wear loose trousers that can easily be rolled up.

CHAPTER 16

My primary treatments

There are a vast number of treatments that can help reduce and heal pain. Over the years, I've trained in several forms of therapy to complement my work as an osteopath so that I can treat my clients in the best way, straight away, rather than sending them to another practitioner – I want a wide-ranging arsenal that I can deploy immediately. This is key when discussing good therapy, and there's no reason why there can't be a combination of several of the treatments listed below in the same session. It has never made sense to me to examine a client, use mobilization, and then book them in for an appointment in a week's time for a massage, and then the week after that for cold laser therapy. A lot of these therapies complement each other, so why shouldn't I use all three in the same session?

My aim has always been to provide the maximum relief with the minimum discomfort, and I have adapted my methods over the years to achieve this. None of these therapies should leave a patient in pain or significant discomfort – this shouldn't be another instance of 'no pain, no gain'. I learnt early on in my career that it's not only about dealing with the problem, but also about making the client feel really good afterwards. It's important to keep this in mind when being treated by a professional.

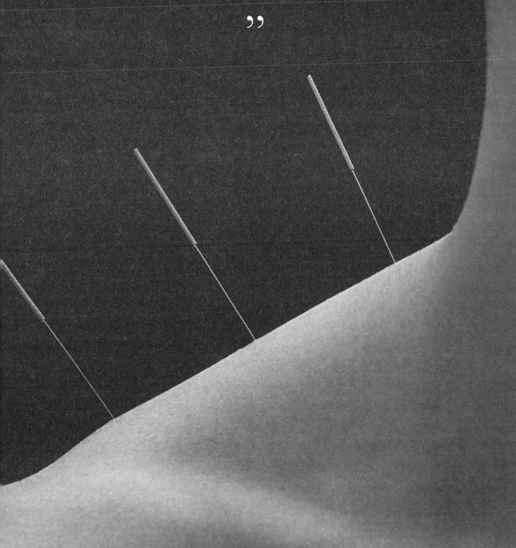

" "

My aim is to provide the maximum relief
with the minimum discomfort.

" "

Throughout this chapter I will explore the treatments that I use in my own practice or of which I have a good working knowledge. They are a combination of mainstream healthcare and complementary or alternative practices. Most people naturally lean to either one side or the other when it comes to treatment, but I believe in a mixture of the two as they often balance each other.

CLICKING AND MOBILIZATION

Clicking is used when there is a restriction of movement in a joint. Clicking is also known as manipulation, cracking, or high-velocity thrusts. A therapist will use a short thrust to 'click' the joint and restore its full function. If a joint is out of sync, then this often causes pain and inflammation of the area and clicking can help alleviate this. All your joints can be clicked, but it is used on mostly the neck and back. A rib can also be clicked back into place if it has been dislodged.

PATIENT FILES: CLICKING

Amelie came to see me about her knee, and I noticed that one of her shoulders was slightly raised. I asked her about it, and she told me that for over ten years it had often been sore and she experienced more intense shoulder pain when carrying a bag. She had been for a few massages and the pain then lessened for a bit, but would then return a few days later. I examined her back and she was very tight around her neck and her spine was slightly raised. When I pressed on the tip of her first rib it was tender on one side but not the other. I knew then that her first rib, which is up near the top of the shoulder, was out of sync. I spent some time loosening the tissues around it while explaining that the only way to resolve the problem was to click the rib. She agreed to this and when it was done there was such a loud noise that she gasped – it was very far out of sync – and she felt an instant release of tension in the muscles around her shoulders and upper back. The shape of her spine and shoulder returned to normal and she no longer had pain in her shoulder and back.

It sounds obvious – but still needs stating – that clicking is something that should only ever be done by someone who is fully trained as damage can easily be caused. There are over 100 clicking techniques and I learnt about them when I was training to be an osteopath. For the first two years of study, I learnt about how a healthy joint with full mobility should feel. Later in the course, the tutor showed us the technique for clicking a particular joint and we went off in pairs and practised on each other. This was only after we had been studying anatomy for at least two years – we knew the exact part we were trying to trigger just by looking at the surface of the skin.

MYTH BUSTERS

The noise produced when clicking is not actually the bone rubbing against another bone, but the release of gas in the joint – this is the same for all clicking. Cracking our knuckles is also a type of clicking. We've often been told that cracking our knuckles can lead to arthritis, but there's evidence that this is untrue, although it may damage the bones and joints in other ways.

It's important that any tight muscles around a joint are loosened up before you have a joint clicked and, in my opinion, a therapist should always ask for permission from the client to use clicking. The best method of clicking is when it is a precise movement to a joint that does the least damage to the surrounding tissue. Many people think that the quality of the 'click' is how loud it is, or how many cracks they hear, but this isn't necessarily the case. The classic 'popping' or 'clicking' noise is produced by a release of gas in the joint, but it's not an open-air concert – louder doesn't always mean better.

Even one session of clicking can be beneficial, and I often see it restore movement back to a joint that has previously been severely restricted. But it's not something that should be done every week; if the joint is constantly coming out of sync, then the surrounding tissue needs to be strengthened, so that it keeps the joint in the correct position. Clicking is therefore not a long-term solution if it needs to be done repeatedly to the same joint. It should also be combined with massage to ensure that the muscles around the joint are healthy and flexible.

Clicking requires a high degree of skill. There are some people who have only completed a rushed intensive course over a weekend, so it's always best to ask around for a recommendation, or consider if the practitioner is well established. I've had several patients come to me because clicking has been done incorrectly and caused an injury. I usually recommend that you go to an osteopath or

"CLICKING REQUIRES A HIGH DEGREE OF SKILL."

chiropractor for clicking, although some physiotherapists have done postgraduate courses in it, and they also have the formal training in anatomy to be able to do it properly. A case-history form should also always be done before clicking, as it's not a suitable treatment for all patients.

Before trying clicking, a therapist should usually try to manipulate the joint back into the right place through another technique called 'mobilization'. This is a much slower and gentler motion, but is still very effective at restoring mobility to a joint. My general rule is to try mobilization first and work around the soft tissues before moving on to clicking, but only if it is needed.

There are many YouTube videos on how to click your own neck, but I cannot stress this strongly enough: never try to click your own neck! Even if, miraculously, you have the right technique, it takes a skilled practitioner to work out which facet joint needs clicking, and you could be clicking away happily at the wrong one and causing damage to a perfectly healthy joint. There are also so many arteries running around your spine that you could damage one of these, which could lead to a stroke – there have been recorded cases of this happening. If you can't afford to see a private practitioner, then your doctor should be able to refer you to a physiotherapist through the NHS.

DRY NEEDLING AND ELECTROACUPUNCTURE

Dry needling is something I use on my patients most weeks. It's also known as 'medical acupuncture' and is considered the 'Western' version of acupuncture. If you came into my treatment room when I was using it, you might think that I was carrying out acupuncture as the two look very similar – several fine needles are inserted into a specifically chosen area of the body. But this is where the similarities end as the placement of the needles is decided by two very different systems.

With acupuncture, the needle is usually inserted into an area of the body that is not the direct site of the injury, as the practitioner aims to balance a flow of energy through the body. There is more information on acupuncture in Chapter 17.

Dry needling, or medical acupuncture, is used directly where the source of the pain or injury is. It isn't about balancing any type of energy, and instead it tries to encourage the body to heal the site of the injury. It's called 'dry' needling as nothing is injected into the body. When the fine needle is inserted under the skin, it provides a stimulus that sends a signal to the brain that there has been an injury to the area. The brain then reacts by increasing the blood flow to this specific part, which contains beneficial nutrients, oxygen, and chemicals that will aid healing. Put simply, dry needling reminds the brain to heal an area of the body.

> **"DRY NEEDLING REMINDS THE BRAIN TO HEAL AN AREA OF THE BODY."**

The National Institute for Health and Care Excellence (NICE), which provides guidelines for the NHS, recently approved acupuncture and dry needling for the treatment of chronic pain in a 'traditional Chinese or Western acupuncture system' (NICE Guidelines NG193, 7 April 2021). The NHS also approved them for the treatment of chronic tension-type headaches and migraines.

The beauty of dry needling comes from its precision. The needles are so fine that the practitioner can direct them to a very specific location. Massage can also help improve circulation and healing, but

DRY
NEEDLING

only to a more generalized area, and therefore can potentially cause damage to the surrounding tissue if it is torn. The two therapies often complement each other and I regularly use them together.

In addition to encouraging healing, I also use dry needling to release tension in muscles. When I am examining a client, I make a note of any tight muscles. Then, when it comes to treatment, I place several fine needles in the muscle for either a few seconds or several minutes, depending on what I think it needs. When I first began practising dry needling, I used to sometimes leave the needles in for twenty minutes. I'm more experienced now and find that combining dry needling with massaging the area before and afterwards works just as well, and it's less likely to cause negative side effects such as soreness. For me, it has always been about devising methods to obtain the maximum effect with the minimum discomfort for the patient. When I take the needle out, I can usually see a distinct difference in the tone of the muscle.

Another method I use is to insert and remove the needle repeatedly from the muscle, and when this is done it's normal for it to twitch. I usually ask the patient to touch the muscle before and after the treatment so they can feel the difference in the muscle tone for themselves.

In my experience, dry needling works well on the back, particularly when there are problems with the discs. The area I use it on most commonly is the upper trapezius muscles in the back, as they carry a lot of tension due to stress and posture. I also use it a lot for plantar fasciitis, which is a painful strain injury at the bottom of the foot. The

ELECTROAC

skin around there is quite tough, so it can be one of those rare occasions when it might be a little painful when the needles are inserted. Dry needling also works well for joint problems and bruising of the bone as the tip of the needle can be placed directly on the bone. Needles inserted into the back of the neck can also help alleviate headaches.

Electroacupuncture is something I also regularly use. The electrical current provides an increased stimulus in a shorter amount of time than dry needling. This is beneficial because the less time the needle is in place, then the less chance there is of there being soreness afterwards. With electroacupuncture, the needles are inserted into the treatment area and then small crocodile clips are attached to the ends of the needles and a small current is sent through them.

With all types of acupuncture and dry needling, the needles should be sterile and only used once before being thrown away. Usually, patients need a course of dry needling but should feel the benefit from only one session if this is all they can afford. There are different thicknesses of needles and, with a skilled therapist, you shouldn't feel any pain when the needle is inserted. There is a real skill to minimizing the pain by pinching the skin together when inserting the needle. When I trained, I used to spend hours practising on myself so I could insert the needle without any discomfort. It was only then that I started practising on other people such as my family and colleagues. Very occasionally, the needle might hurt even with a skilled practitioner where the skin is tough, such as the heel of the foot, but this should be rare.

JPUNCTURE

Acupuncture and dry needling are generally considered very safe. However, I have heard of cases where an unqualified or unskilled therapist has punctured a patient's lung because they used a long needle and entered it directly downwards into the back, rather than at an angle. For this reason, it's essential that the practitioner has a good knowledge of surface anatomy (see box, page 301), so they know by sight and feel where the lungs and other organs are, along with the blood vessels and main nerves. Therefore, you should make sure that the person performing the treatment is qualified and experienced. Nowadays, you can go on a weekend course and say

> "MAKE SURE THE PERSON PERFORMING THE TREATMENT IS QUALIFIED AND EXPERIENCED."

that you are qualified in dry needling as long as you are able to obtain insurance. There's no national register of licensed practitioners in the UK, so I would recommend looking for an osteopath, chiropractor, or physiotherapist who does dry needling.

NON-INVASIVE TISSUE-REPAIR TREATMENTS

There are several non-invasive treatments that help heal damaged tissue that require specialist equipment and I will run through the ones that I believe have the best outcomes. I regularly use all of them, apart from ultrasound. As with all treatments, it's important to go to a therapist who is trained, has the right equipment, and is experienced in using it. I would also recommend seeing a qualified osteopath, chiropractor, or physiotherapist when it comes to these treatments.

All of the following treatments are particularly useful when a client is in such acute or chronic pain that they feel sensitive to touch. In those cases, these therapies that use either light, sound waves, or electrical currents can ease their pain without making them more uncomfortable in the process.

ULTRASOUND

Most people think of ultrasound as a method of scanning, but it is used as a treatment as well. Gel is applied to the skin and then the small ultrasound head is placed on the area that needs treating. It uses sound waves to help with circulation, thus reducing pain and increasing the rate of healing.

Ultrasound is the grandad of these non-invasive tissue-repair systems. One of the reasons I don't use it is because it was popular around twenty or thirty years ago, but times have moved on. It's still an effective treatment to aid healing but, in my opinion, the following treatments have overtaken it.

COLD LASER THERAPY

Cold laser therapy utilizes a frequency of low-level laser light that I have found to be very effective. It is still considered an experimental treatment, but more studies are being carried out as it's a relatively new treatment. Athletes use it regularly, but it's not currently available on the NHS. The laser is contained in a small hand-held device, and it's classed as 'cold' as it won't cut or burn through tissue, unlike the much stronger lasers that are used in surgery. The laser stimulates tissue repair and circulation, all the things we know are needed in the healing process. It can desensitize a patient to pain and help with removing waste products from the site.

PATIENT FILES: ACHILLES TENDON STRAIN

Dan was training for his third marathon when he started to get pain around his Achilles tendon on both sides of his leg. He first came to see me when it was so tender that he wouldn't let anyone touch it. As I was unable to touch his calves to treat them, I used cold laser therapy. Afterwards, it was less tender and I could even pinch the skin around the tendon. He had a course of cold laser therapy and this relieved his pain.

I've seen the best results when treating the knee joint and it also helps with muscle tears. It's particularly good on arthritic knees.

I have a class-four laser. Members of the public can buy less powerful ones, but they are not as effective as the ones that a qualified professional will use. The treatment doesn't hurt, but there is a slight warmth on the skin. The average time that the laser should be used on a body part is five to ten minutes. It shouldn't be used over areas that are tattooed as it can heat the ink up and cause pain.

SHOCKWAVE

Extracorporeal Shockwave Therapy is a treatment for acute and chronic pain that has been around for several decades. It is available on the NHS, as well as from private practitioners. It is clinically proven to help increase the blood flow and the body's healing process. A hand-held device sends sound waves into a targeted area of the body. The treatment can be a little uncomfortable as the sound waves feel like pulses, but it shouldn't be painful.

Shockwave therapy is quick and effective, and the results are usually immediately noticeable. I find that shockwave treatment is particularly effective on tendons, especially the Achilles tendon, and it can be used on bones as well. When I was working with the Olympic team, I used it on the junction where the muscle and the tendon meet, particularly around the hamstring. It can also help break down scar tissue.

> "SHOCKWAVE THERAPY IS PARTICULARLY EFFECTIVE ON TENDONS."

TECAR THERAPY

Tecar is another relatively new therapy in the UK, and therefore hasn't yet undergone the clinical trials that shockwave therapy has had. It originated in Italy and Spain and is common across Europe. It is used by athletes and Premiership football teams, but isn't available on the NHS. It's still pretty rare in the UK and I'm one of a handful of therapists who use it here. Every week I get a call from someone who has just moved from Italy, or who has an Italian uncle who swears by Tecar therapy, so they are trying to find someone who can provide it.

Tecar therapy delivers an electrical current through a hand-held device where you can change the size of the head for precision. A gel is applied to a mat on which the client lies down, and which completes the circuit for the electrical current. It can get a little messy at times as the mat is covered in gel. The therapy can be used to reduce pain and inflammation and decrease the healing time. It helps to warm up the ligaments, tendons, and bones, which is a pleasant sensation.

"TECAR IS BETTER FOR TREATING A VARIETY OF CONDITIONS."

I use Tecar therapy more than shockwave therapy and it's a good all-rounder for treating muscles. It can be used on joints as well, but I tend to use it on muscles for either acute or chronic pain. It can treat the top levels of the muscles and the deeper tissues such as tendons, so it is better for treating a variety of conditions than the other non-invasive treatments.

TRANSCUTANEOUS ELECTRICAL NERVE STIMULATION (TENS) MACHINE

A TENS machine is something that I often recommend that my clients invest in, particularly if they are recovering from a traumatic injury or are training very hard for a sporting event. It uses a mild electrical current, and the machines have become quite advanced over the years. Some of them are wireless and I normally use them on a muscle that has lost its size and depth. There are many settings on an advanced TENS machine and they can help:

- Reduce pain in muscles and joints, particularly in the lower back and knee

- Reduce muscle tightness and tension

- Build muscle

- Improve circulation

- Lymphatic draining

- Recovery from bruising

- Recovery between workout sessions or other activities that overwork the muscles

MASSAGE

It may not come as a surprise to learn that there are records of massage having been used for thousands of years. It is believed to have originated in India, China, and Egypt, and the first book on massage techniques was written in China around 2700 BC.

Massage has more benefits than just being relaxing – it can reduce tension and soreness in muscles and stimulates blood flow. It also isn't just for the back or limbs. I regularly use visceral massage, which is a gentle massage of the abdomen, as it can help with constipation and problems with the gut. Massage is one of my most used therapies and I usually begin a session with it. I massage an area and use the time to assess the muscles, tendons, and joints with my hands – a way of combining diagnosis with treatment.

I would like to start by saying that massage should feel nice. You shouldn't come out of a session feeling pummelled and worse than

PATIENT FILES: MASSAGE

Michael, who worked as a chauffeur, came to see me with pain in his lower back and restless legs. After examining him I realized the muscles in his legs weren't tight so I massaged the surface muscles lightly, trying to encourage the circulation of blood and drainage. A different massaging technique was then needed in his lower back, where he had deep muscles that were in spasm and very tight, and it required firm pressure to loosen and relax them.

when you first went in — aches and pains afterwards do not mean that you've had a more beneficial therapy session. Equally, you shouldn't feel like you've just been lightly tickled and so wonder if you just paid a lot of money to lie down on a table with a hole cut out for your head.

There should be a degree of pleasant aching afterwards, especially if you don't have regular massages and your muscles need a lot of work. The point of massage is to release the tension in the muscles that are tight, so that if you run your hand over them, it's a smooth ride and not bumpy. At the beginning, it might be a bit painful, but as the treatment goes on, the pain should lessen. At the same time the client should be relaxed as the massage helps release endorphins, which won't happen if they are tensed up waiting for the next time the massage therapist attacks a knot in their shoulder. After a massage you should leave the table feeling good about yourself and energized.

> "THE POINT OF MASSAGE IS TO RELEASE THE TENSION IN THE MUSCLES."

However, I also have a small bone to pick with massage and the way it is sometimes advertised. We live in a time when, from the massage menu, you must choose whether you have a deep-tissue massage, sports massage, or Swedish massage, when they're all effectively the same as they just massage the deeper layers of the muscle. Or we think a lighter massage might be more beneficial as it will be more relaxing, so we pick that one instead. There might even be several names of massage techniques that are thrown into the mix that we are not familiar with, such as tapotement, petrissage, or effleurage, and we believe that we might even have to choose between those as well. When faced with all these options, what should we do?

In my opinion, the answer is that we put ourselves in the hands of a skilled therapist who will choose for us. It shouldn't be the case that the responsibility for selecting the right treatment is transferred to the client, when really the deepness and techniques used during the massage should change depending on each muscle, what condition the client's body is in, and the areas that need working on. Massage is massage, and the therapist should know when to go deep or when to be gentle with a muscle. A true therapist, and there are plenty of them out there, will trust what their hands are telling them.

The benefits of massage are immeasurable. I use it in conjunction with many other therapies and it's a rare session in which I don't use it at all. The benefits from massage can be felt in only one session, but in an ideal world you will have regular massages, every four weeks if you can, as massage prevents injuries and is a good investment because of this. If you can't afford this, then there's more in Chapter 21 about massage techniques, if you want to do this with a partner or friend. One thing to remember is that you shouldn't have a firm, deep massage a day or two before a sporting event because it can make you more susceptible to injuries when your muscles are repairing.

If you have a skilled therapist, all areas of the muscle should be treated – the sides are often ignored. Also, if you've got lower-back pain the glutes will be tight and these should be massaged. Some therapists won't work on the buttocks, but these muscles are very important when it comes to lower-back pain. Another common occurrence is that the shoulders will be massaged and the therapist might comment that they are knotty, but often the bumps are the ribs, which go right up the back to the area in line with the top of the shoulders. A good knowledge of surface anatomy is therefore useful. The whole body should also be covered in the session rather than concentrating on a couple of specific areas.

There are also some parts of the body that will naturally feel tight such as the iliotibial (IT) band, which is a length of thick tissue that runs from the outside of your thighs to the knee. It's connective tissue so it should be tight, and therefore doesn't need to be pummelled. Heat is also good for loosening muscles so warm hands and a warm room are ideal.

THE BENEFITS OF MASSAGE ARE
IMMEAS

PAINKILLERS

How many of us look at the back of a box of painkillers to check the side effects before popping them in our mouths? I talked about painkillers in Chapter 2, but it's good to reiterate that painkillers aren't ideal for long-term use, other than in cases of palliative care. They'll become less effective as time goes on, and there is a serious risk of addiction to opioids.

The National Institute for Health and Care Excellence (NICE), which provides guidelines for the NHS, has recently changed its advice on prescribing painkillers to new sufferers of chronic primary pain (i.e. pain lasting over three months where the source of the pain is not known):

"

People with chronic primary pain should not be started on commonly used drugs including paracetamol, non-steroidal anti-inflammatory drugs, benzodiazepines or opioids. This is because there is little or no evidence that they make any difference to people's quality of life, pain or psychological distress, but they can cause harm, including possible addiction.
(NICE news release, Guidelines NG193, 7 April 2021).

"

Instead, NICE advises that a care and support plan is supplied; and treatments, including exercise programmes, psychological therapies, and acupuncture, are recommended.

However, in the short term, painkillers can be beneficial when the underlying cause of the pain is being treated. It's always important to remember, when taking painkillers, not to overexert the area that

URABLE

is causing the pain while you can't feel it. When we take painkillers, we effectively numb the signals that our bodies are trying to send, and therefore we might cause more damage if we can't receive these messages. When taking painkillers, it's important to speak to your doctor if you are taking other medications because it can be dangerous to mix medications. Here are the most common painkillers and what they are used to treat:

PARACETAMOL

This is a general painkiller, which we probably all have in our cupboards, and is designed to treat mild to moderate pain. It's used for headaches and muscle aches, but can also treat high temperatures as well. It rarely causes side effects if it is taken correctly, but there is a limit on how many pills can be taken daily, so if you build up a resistance to it and are at the maximum dosage, you can't increase it.

NON-STEROIDAL ANTI-INFLAMMATORY DRUGS (NSAIDS)

Non-steroidal anti-inflammatory drugs (NSAIDs) are another type of painkiller that we often have in our cupboards, and include ibuprofen and aspirin. These are both used to treat inflammation by reducing the hormones that produce swelling, which is a common outcome of a tissue injury. Ibuprofen is more commonly used for anti-inflammatory purposes as it is better at treating pain than aspirin. Ibuprofen is not recommended for long-term use unless advised by a doctor, and it has more common side effects than paracetamol, including stomach problems, kidney problems and, ironically, headaches.

OPIOIDS

Opioids are typically used to treat moderate to severe pain and must be prescribed by a doctor, although co-codamol can be bought without a prescription. Co-codamol is a mixture of paracetamol and codeine and used to treat migraines, headaches, and general muscle pain when paracetamol and ibuprofen have not worked. Opioids also include codeine and morphine and are not recommended for long-term use, except with terminal illnesses, as there is a risk of addiction. The side effects of co-codamol can include nausea, constipation, and dizziness.

PERFORMANCE THERAPY

Performance therapy is something that has been used for athletes for several years, but it is starting to become more common in gyms in America now. Performance therapy is a quick pit stop for therapy, usually when someone is in the middle of exercising. I used it a lot when I was a therapist for track and field competitions. I would stand on the sidelines wherever the training was taking place and watch an athlete's movements to see if a muscle was beginning to get tight. They would then come over for treatment and I would usually loosen up a muscle to help improve their performance. It's all about a quick repair, so they might need a click, a stretch, a release of a muscle, or an active release, which is pressing on a muscle and using the area or the limb as a lever. Then they would return to training, and I'd watch to see if it had helped. If it hadn't, then I knew we'd need to do more work on the area.

> "IT'S A QUICK PIT STOP FOR THERAPY WHEN SOMEONE IS EXERCISING."

Nowadays, I use performance therapy when a client is training in a gym. When they are doing a bicep curl, I might notice that there is something wrong with their shoulder and I'll quickly loosen it up.

The reason I'm mentioning this here is because it soon won't just be for elite athletes. In America, gyms now often have employees who watch the people training and will quickly use a massage gun on them if they think a muscle is getting tight. As with most things in America, they usually cross the ocean to us, so I think this will start happening in UK gyms in the next few years.

It's also something that you will hopefully incorporate into your own daily routine. Both the set of stretches at the beginning of your day, or the massage gun or foam roller you use during the day, are a form of performance therapy – that is, it's a quick session where you are offsetting any potential problems that could happen later.

CHAPTER 17

Other treatment options

This chapter covers treatments that either I am trained in, but don't use every week, or have experienced several times and believe are beneficial. Most of them fall under 'alternative' and 'complementary' therapies.

Strong feelings about complementary and alternative medicine on both sides of the camps exist. Some call them 'pseudoscience', whereas others believe in them with every fibre of their being.

In recent years the NHS has slowly started to explore the benefits of complementary and alternative therapies. It may surprise you to learn that the NHS classes osteopathy and chiropractic practitioners under these titles, despite them using similar methods to physiotherapy. However, in the UK, osteopathy and chiropractic treatments are the only complementary and alternative therapies that are regulated in the same way as conventional medicine.

We live in a time when statements need to be backed by research, and this is often where alternative medicines fall short. The ability to conduct clinical trials that satisfy the rigorous testing the scientific community requires is the hurdle at which alternative therapies often fail. When these clinical trials are conducted there needs to be a test group that is given a treatment that feels similar but is known not to be

"
Strong feelings about complimentary
and alternative medicine on both sides
of the camps exist.
"

beneficial – that is, a placebo. The outcomes of the placebo are then weighed against the outcomes of the treatment.

The first problem is to find a suitable placebo; it's not as simple as testing a medicine where you can replace a new painkiller with a sugar pill. The second problem is that people will sometimes feel a benefit from something even if it isn't helping them, which is commonly known as the 'placebo effect'. This is referred to a lot when studies are conducted on alternative therapies as a reason for justifying unexpected positive results. It really is a circular problem – a therapy must show a benefit and any benefit it shows is often explained away by the placebo effect.

As a therapist, I am always learning and open to ideas that are new to me. I can always be a better therapist. I've been very lucky to have visited other parts of the world and experienced different treatments, as well as learning from other Olympic teams about how they approach therapy. My view has always been that I want my patients to get from A to Z, and if a complementary or alternative therapy helps with this process, and the client feels a benefit, then it should be used alongside conventional treatment. I honestly believe that we often need a mixture of conventional and complementary therapies to achieve the best results.

> "I WANT PATIENTS TO GET FROM A TO Z, AND IF AN ALTERNATIVE THERAPY HELPS THEN IT SHOULD BE USED."

My aim has never been to force my opinions on people, as I respect that there will always be differing viewpoints. I can therefore only say what I have experienced with the following treatments and what my clients have told me. In my practice, I always use a new treatment or device on myself several times before I consider using it on clients. Some of the following treatments I use in my own practice and others I have experienced and found to be beneficial. I'll then let you decide for yourself if you want to try any of them.

When looking for a practitioner I would always advise starting with a recommendation from a family member or friend and checking if the practitioner is registered with either the Complementary and Natural Healthcare Council (www.cnhc.org.uk) or the Federation of Holistic Therapists (fht.org.uk). Registration with either of these bodies is voluntary, but is a good place to start when finding the right therapist for you.

ACUPUNCTURE AND ACUPRESSURE

Acupuncture has been around for several thousand years, and it's generally agreed that it originates from China. The belief behind acupuncture is that energy called *qi* (pronounced 'chee') flows through the body. There are twelve principal pathways of qi, which are called *meridians*. Each meridian is associated with one of our organs and other bodily functions. The meridians flow through a specific area of the body, but don't follow the same routes as blood vessels or nerves. Acupuncture is used for pain relief, general ailments, or to target specific problems such as addiction to cigarettes. The practitioner uses a needle and places it into the meridian to try and balance the flow of qi. The place where the needle is inserted rarely corresponds with the area that needs treating. For example, a therapist might insert a needle into a patient's hand to treat the large intestine or the ear for someone who wants to quit smoking.

"EACH MERIDIAN IS ASSOCIATED WITH ONE OF OUR ORGANS AND OTHER BODILY FUNCTIONS."

Acupuncture is used in doctors' surgeries, pain clinics, and hospices throughout the UK and has recently been approved by the National Institute for Health and Care Excellence (NICE), alongside dry needling, for the treatment of chronic pain, as well as to treat chronic tension-type headaches and migraines.

Acupressure is often used with acupuncture and works on a similar principle, but without the needles. Instead, the therapist presses on the area of the body where the meridian is located.

From my experience, I have found acupuncture and acupressure to be beneficial. I've had it several times and have felt energized afterwards. It has also helped me with lower-back pain, and even once when I had flu. My clients have told me that it has helped them with pain relief and increased their energy; and some also believe that it has helped them conceive.

Acupuncture is sometimes available on the NHS, usually either in a doctor's practice or with a physiotherapist who has been trained in it. If you decide to pay for it privately then always start with a recommendation or try to find out from a therapist how long they have been doing it for and where they qualified.

COLONICS

Colonic irrigation, or colonic hydrotherapy, has been used for at least 2,000 years. It's the practice of inserting a tube into the rectum and then pumping warm water into the colon. The water is then drained back out bringing all the waste products in your bowel with it. The pumping and drainage cycle is done several times while the abdomen is massaged. There's no mess or odour, and those who advocate it believe that it helps improve digestion and weight loss, and alleviates constipation.

"THEY WANTED TO PUT A TUBE UP WHERE?"

I had my first colonic at a health retreat in Chiang Mai in Thailand, when I was 24 years old. I was with my mum who suggested (forced!) me to have one. I was very reluctant – they wanted to put a tube up where? But afterwards I felt lighter, less bloated, and as if the pressure had been taken away from my lower back.

I now try to have two colonics a year if I can. You have to see a private practitioner for this, so ask for a recommendation and check online reviews as well. Colonics are no substitution for keeping your bowel healthy and you can do this by:

"COLONICS ARE NO SUBSTITUTION FOR KEEPING YOUR BOWEL HEALTHY."

- Drinking enough water to regulate your digestive system. Most clients I see with colon issues such as constipation don't drink enough water.

- Eat a high-fibre diet.

- Drink probiotics.

- Drink smoothies or juices.

CRANIOSACRAL THERAPY

Craniosacral therapy, or 'cranial osteopathy', uses light pressure from a therapist's hands to gently manipulate the skull, pelvis, and spine to treat various disorders in the body. The theory behind it is that manipulation of the skull can affect and balance the fluid surrounding the spinal cord. The difference between cranial osteopathy and craniosacral therapy depends on who is practising it and where they were taught. The former is performed by an osteopath and the latter by any other therapist such as a chiropractor, massage therapist, or a therapist who specializes in this therapy. I was taught cranial osteopathy as part of my degree and spent hours practising on another student's head, trying to feel the different cranial bones.

Cranial osteopathy and craniosacral therapy are very gentle and because of this they are commonly used to treat babies, the elderly, or people who cannot face rigorous treatment. I use it occasionally in my practice, such as with a baby who isn't sleeping or eating very well, and afterwards the parents have told me that these both improved. I've also used it lower down on the sacrum for a client who had lower-back pain and couldn't stand for it to be touched; afterwards he was less tender. I've also had feedback from my clients that it helps with sinus issues.

CUPPING

Cupping has become very fashionable in the last few years, but it has been around for a few thousand years. It originates from Egypt, China, and the Middle East. Cups can be applied anywhere on the body but are commonly used on the back, shoulders, and buttocks. Several cups are used in turn, and they look like a tumbler glass, depending on what material they are made from. I use glass or bamboo cups, but there are plastic ones as well.

The idea is that the suction from the cups improves circulation and draws the blood to the surface of the skin. I've found that it also works well to ease tight muscles and complements massage for this reason. Some of my clients have reported that it has helped fade stretch marks if used soon after giving birth and others have said that it helps with sluggish bowels when used on the lower back. I also use it as a diagnostic tool to see if a patient is dehydrated, or if there are a lot of toxins in their body. It's commonly used by athletes despite there not being many controlled studies on its benefits.

> "THE IDEA IS THE SUCTION FROM THE CUPS IMPROVES CIRCULATION."

The client lies down and I quickly place a flame inside the cup, which sucks the oxygen out of it and creates a vacuum. The cup is then placed on the area that I'm treating. The skin is drawn up into the cup and the surface reddens as blood flows into the area. The intensity of the cupping pressure is governed by the length of time the flame is left in the cup. Plastic cups can have a pump on them so there isn't any need to have the flame.

Even though a flame is used the cup doesn't (and shouldn't) feel hot for the client. But it will often leave a red circular mark on the body from the suction – this was famously shown when the Olympic swimmer Michael Phelps was photographed in 2016 – but these should fade after a few days to a couple of weeks. Therefore, if you do decide to have cupping, please have a think about what you will be doing over the next couple of weeks as you might not want large red marks across your back in your wedding photos! I've also seen cases where the pressure of the vacuum has been too high and led to blisters, which obviously isn't an acceptable outcome. As with all the treatments, try to find someone who is experienced and has been recommended to you.

From my experience, cupping is very relaxing and a great stress reliever. Therefore, I think it's beneficial to most people just as a therapeutic treatment.

PILATES

Pilates has been around for over a hundred years and its aim is to strengthen the body, with a particular emphasis on posture, balance, flexibility, and core strength. Pilates was developed in the early twentieth century by Joseph Pilates, who was born in Germany in 1880. Always interested in different methods of exercising, he was one of the first therapists to mix Eastern and Western ideologies. When he was in his early thirties he moved to Britain. During the First World War, he was interned because of his German origins, and it was during this time of imprisonment that he developed the exercise regime that would later be known as Pilates. It is suitable for all fitness levels and ages, and can be done with a piece of equipment called a 'reformer', or simply on a mat using your body weight for resistance.

"I RECOMMEND PILATES TO CLIENTS IF THEY HAVE LOWER BACK PAIN."

Clients often ask me if they should be doing yoga or Pilates. I regularly recommend Pilates to clients if they have lower-back pain as it can help stabilize the area where there is a weakness or discomfort. I've found that it also helps with problems with pelvis alignment, which is a common issue linked to lower-back pain, as it helps improve the relationship of the lower back, pelvis, and hip.

I think that when it comes to both yoga and Pilates, the instructor is really important. Any feedback that you get when in the class can help prevent injuries. It's common in a class environment for everyone to be at different levels, so don't expect your body to be capable of what the person on the next mat is doing. Instead, try to focus on your own progress. Pilates isn't suitable for people with certain medical conditions and therefore you should provide details of your medical history before you begin. Yoga and Pilates shouldn't hurt – there might be a gentle aching afterwards but during the class you shouldn't feel any pain. Like all things, listen to your body. If something doesn't feel right, then stop.

TOK SEN

Tok Sen is a form of massage that has been practised in Thailand for over 5,000 years. It was developed by monks who used a wooden hammer and small wedge from the wood of a tamarind tree. 'Tok' means to hit or hammer, and 'sen' means energy pathways. The hammer and wedge are used to tap rhythmically on muscles, tendons, and ligaments to stimulate the area, helping to release energy within the body to promote good health and wellbeing. Like all massage, it is aimed to relax the body and mind, but I have found that it can also relieve pain and tension in the body. Advocates for the treatment say that it can help the immune system, increase circulation, and improve alignment.

> "THE HAMMER AND WEDGE ARE USED TO TAP RHYTHMICALLY ON MUSCLES, TENDONS, AND LIGAMENTS."

I first came across Tok Sen on a visit to Thailand. I had a few sessions and found it beneficial, so I eventually decided to train in it. I normally use it on athletes as it activates the muscles and awakens the nerves – there are many cases where I've tapped around the buttock muscles and there has been more movement in the hips afterwards. I combine it with a general massage and use it around the pelvis, lower back, and buttocks. The reason I mainly use it on athletes is because they are so strong in these three areas. I often use it as an alternative to dry needling if I can't do that at the time of treatment.

YOGA

Yoga is an ancient form of exercise that has been around for 5,000 years and originated in India. It involves holding poses that aid flexibility while concentrating on your breathing. It can help with meditation as well. I have found that it helps with tuning into your body and is a calming therapy that aids general wellbeing.

Traditionally, yoga would be done on a one-to-one basis, but in modern times it is more common to practise it in a large class environment. I see quite a few clients who have injured themselves during a yoga class, so it's always good to be aware of your body's limitations. If you find a particular pose difficult, it might be better to do a couple of stretches instead, as you might have a structural reason that means that you can't bend a certain way. If it's a natural part of your body, it's not going to function the same as everyone else's. That's not a weakness; it's just how you've been built.

"YOGA INJURIES ARE COMMON, SO IT'S ALWAYS GOOD TO BE AWARE OF YOUR BODY'S LIMITATIONS."

There are all sorts of classes available now, from traditional methods of yoga to hot yoga. It's also freely available on the internet and is even taught in schools. You also don't necessarily need to go to a yoga class to enjoy the benefits of it. Something simple like the Child's Pose first thing in the morning can help awaken your muscles. Clients tell me that it helps relieve stress as the breathing techniques relax their mind, as well as incorporating all the benefits of gentle exercise.

PART FOUR

Reset and Body Reform

CHAPTER 18

Stress and
anxiety

Let's turn our attention to stress and anxiety, because both conditions, when left unchecked, manifest in the body as pain. They are another signal that something isn't quite right. I would say that 90 per cent of the clients I see have lingering symptoms of stress and anxiety that are so chronic that they have physical consequences. Some of them don't even feel stressed, but their muscles are tight in their neck, shoulders, or chest, and they don't recognize this as a symptom of stress. Or they have headaches, digestion issues, or frequent illnesses and don't link these to stress either. There is now evidence that long-term stress has such a detrimental effect on our system that it can even reduce life expectancy.

Before we can tackle stress and anxiety, we need to understand it so we can recognize it, because stress is a source of pain and, as we now know, pain should never be ignored.

"
Long-term stress can even
reduce life expectancy.
"

WHAT IS STRESS?

Stress has managed to get itself a bad reputation in the past few decades. 'I'm so stressed!' 'I can't take any more of this stress!' 'He is stressing me out!' We all say things like this as we rush between meetings, eating on the go, rarely catching a glimpse of sunlight from our offices in the winter months. We live in a fast-paced world that demands we keep up or we will be replaced, let go, or forgotten. And to keep up we must cram every minute with 'more'. More meetings, more social occasions, more calls, more events, more work trips, more exercise classes, more retreats, more friends, and definitely more life-changing experiences.

> "IN ITS PUREST FORM, AND JUST LIKE PAIN, STRESS IS A LIFESAVER."

Most of us recognize negative stress, but perhaps we don't know what stress does and how there can be a positive side to stress as well.

In its purest form, and just like pain, stress is a lifesaver. It is the body's response to either a real or perceived danger that triggers a biological response within the body.

Let me take you back to a time when we set off in the mornings to gather supplies. We walked for six hours a day, occasionally pausing to scoop up firewood or stretching to pluck the highest blackberries from their bushes. As we returned to our shelter for the evening, we held our hand up in greeting to a child who had been waiting patiently for our return since the sun began to set. When we were close to the cave mouth, we heard an unfamiliar noise that made us glance upwards. Dust settled on our hair and our gaze fixed on a fissure in the overhanging rock that was rapidly tracing its way across the stone's underbelly. Our pupils dilated. In a split second our breathing rate hiked up, oxygen flooded into our blood stream, our heart hammered, and the blood vessels

FIGHT

FLIGHT

around it dilated so that essential nutrients, oxygen, and hormones could rush through our body. Our muscles tensed, waiting for the brain to instruct us on how to respond: fight, flight, or freeze. Our brain selected 'flight', and we leapt out of the way as the rock crashed to the ground behind us. It was a rare event, but we survived it.

As we lay there on the ground, our arm still outstretched, our body then had to return itself back to its normal levels – it couldn't stay in this heightened state for long without repercussions. Our heart rate and blood pressure lowered and our breathing returned to normal. Our digestive system, which is not very essential in times of danger, kicked back in again after having been shut down in our earlier heightened state.

All these physical responses were automatic, governed by part of the nervous system. We did not consciously decide that our eyes should dilate, or our blood pressure should lower. If we did, we would lose precious seconds of reaction time. These involuntary responses are controlled by two opposing systems: one that kicks in our 'fight or flight' response and the other that is referred to as the calming 'rest and digest' response.

What we ideally want is a balance between the two, so they both counteract each other when needed and we are not stuck in one or the other. This state of optimal functioning and balance between our autonomic systems is called 'homeostasis' – and this is what we should aim for.

The autonomic system oversees all our involuntary processes such as breathing and heart rate. This system has three parts, the *sympathetic*, the *parasympathetic*, and the *enteric* nervous systems (see Figure 18.1). The *sympathetic* is our alarm that shoots our body into the 'fight or flight' response. It heightens our blood pressure and breathing and reaches nearly every part of our body. The *parasympathetic* has the opposite effect and is described as the 'rest and digest' response. It brings our heart rate back down and slows our breathing. The third part, the *enteric*, governs our digestive system, which is switched off in the sympathetic state and returns in the parasympathetic state.

GOOD AND BAD STRESS

As well as being a lifesaver, stress motivates, focuses, and drives us. If we suddenly receive an email telling us that a project needs to be done by 4.30 p.m., then our stress response kicks in and we get to work. If we remain in our 'rest and digest' response, then this deadline might slide by without us meeting it.

Then, at 4.29 p.m., when we watch the email leave our outbox, we feel energized and proud of ourselves for completing it in time. Our 'rest and digest' system should then flood the body with the hormones and chemicals needed to bring us back down to a neutral state.

But what if we realize we emailed the wrong address? Or we open a letter saying that we've missed a payment on our credit card? Or we have another message saying a new project needs to be completed within two days? Our 'fight or flight' response cranks up again, and those calming periods in between become rarer.

THREE MAIN STRESS HORMONES

There are three main stress hormones: adrenaline, norepinephrine, and cortisol.

1. **ADRENALINE:**
   Adrenaline is the classic 'fight or flight' hormone. It's responsible for increasing your heart rate and supplying instant energy.

2. **NOREPINEPHRINE:**
   Norepinephrine does a similar job to adrenaline. It's an immediate change that also makes you more focused and responsive.

3. **CORTISOL:**
   Cortisol takes longer to produce – several minutes rather than seconds. It supplies more sugar to your blood and shuts down less essential systems in your body, such as digestion.

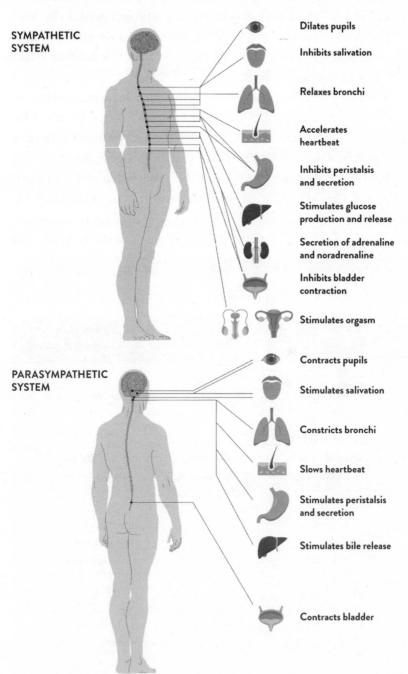

FIG. 18.1
SYMPATHETIC AND PARASYMPATHETIC SYSTEMS

SYMPATHETIC SYSTEM

Dilates pupils

Inhibits salivation

Relaxes bronchi

Accelerates heartbeat

Inhibits peristalsis and secretion

Stimulates glucose production and release

Secretion of adrenaline and noradrenaline

Inhibits bladder contraction

Stimulates orgasm

PARASYMPATHETIC SYSTEM

Contracts pupils

Stimulates salivation

Constricts bronchi

Slows heartbeat

Stimulates peristalsis and secretion

Stimulates bile release

Contracts bladder

This is when good stress becomes harmful – when we are unable to return to that calmer neutral state and are instead constantly being triggered by, and anticipating, the next stressor. It might work for a while and increase our productivity, but at some point things might change. Instead of feeling focused, we'll be jittery and anxious, unable to concentrate on a task and instead circling the room, instinctively trying to burn off excess energy.

When cortisol stays in our body for long periods of time it disrupts our normal systems. Cortisol's job is to shut down certain functions, such as digestion and the immune system, which are seen as less important when facing a life-or-death situation. However, for our general wellbeing, these all need to be fully functioning. We cannot operate as we should with so many compromised functions.

SYMPTOMS OF HIGH CORTISOL LEVELS

Changes to the skin	Thirst	Irregular menstrual cycle
Bladder issues	Mood swings	A puffy face
Changes to your sex drive	Tiredness (including feeling 'tired but wired')	Anxiety
Weight gain	Decreased immunity	Increased blood pressure
	Weakened bones and osteoporosis	

EXAMPLES OF ACUTE AND CHRONIC STRESS

ACUTE STRESS

- You have to give a presentation in front of your team at work.

- You're worried about a big event that's coming up.

- There's bad traffic on the way into work and it looks like you're going to be late.

- You've recently had an argument with your partner.

CHRONIC STRESS

- Bad sleep habits

- Unhealthy relationships or home environment

- Long-term health issues

- A stressful job

- Living in an area with a high crime rate

Like pain, stress can be acute or chronic and this is often guided by outside factors. When a trigger event for stress recurs, the body constantly reacts to it and there is less chance for the 'rest and digest' response to restore us to a balanced state. When considering what is causing stress in our lives, we should start with whether it is a short-term factor or if it is something long term that requires a lifestyle change if we want to tackle it.

WHAT HAPPENS WHEN WE CAN'T RELEASE STRESS?

When we are held in our stress response state for a long period of time it can have a serious effect on our health because our systems are unable to function properly. Even if we enjoy the high of stress it can still create tension in our muscles that will impact on other muscles, tendons, and joints.

If left untreated, we can feel permanently exhausted. It can also interfere with our immune-system responses, which means we are more likely to get ill, causing even more problems for us. Our immune system is a group of cells and organs that defend our bodies from infection. A high temperature is one of our many immune responses and is used to kill invading microbes. If our immune system is constantly overridden by our stress response, it is less able to tackle viruses and bacteria.

Stress has real physical and mental consequences and has been linked to:

- Digestive problems
- Weight gain
- High blood pressure
- Diabetes
- Headaches
- Anxiety
- Depression

- Muscle tension and pain
- Strokes
- Fatigue
- Loss of concentration
- Accelerating the progression of some cancers
- Heart disease

I honestly believe that stress is a silent killer. When so many of our body's precious systems are not able to work properly, because they are

STRESS IS A
SILENT

suppressed by stress hormones, we are creating poor health conditions and leaving ourselves vulnerable to disease and illnesses. Not only this, but we often ignore the other messages our bodies are trying to give to us because we don't have time to listen. My dad was the perfect example of this.

When I was in my late twenties, I went to visit my dad, who had moved to India to work as a civil engineer. He was doing really well in his career, soaring up the ladder, had a PhD – all the evidence of a successful life. As I do for all my friends and family, I offered to treat him as it's my way of looking after people. I noticed straightaway that his mid-back and chest were very stiff as a result of chronic stress and he needed a lifestyle change to address it properly. I mentioned this gently to my dad. Perhaps he could cut down his hours at work? A firm shake of his head let me know that he didn't want to talk about it again.

My dad was always searching. He always wanted more, and he worked all the hours to achieve it. There was no 'reset' button for him. He was always switched on, thinking he was riding the wave of chronic stress, and that he was its master. He didn't have time to eat properly, question why he was suddenly losing weight, or go to the doctor a couple of years later when his skin began turning yellow. He was far too busy to pay attention to that gnawing pain in his abdomen or wonder why it was still there even after his gallbladder had been removed.

It took a diagnosis of pancreatic cancer to stop him in his tracks. All his attention was finally focused on his health, but it was already too late. He died four months later at the age of 61.

I think about my dad a lot and wonder whether he would make the same choices now, knowing what the consequences were. With hindsight, we would often choose differently. My dad is just one example of what can happen when we stop listening to our bodies. Please don't let something similar happen to you.

KILLER

THE EFFECTS OF LONG-
AND SHORT-TERM STRESS

Our body can easily regulate short-term stress as it expects it as a part of life. What it can't function with is long-term stress (see Figure 18.2), so always consider:

BREATHING

- *Short term:* You breathe harder and faster, but breathing should settle quickly once the stressful event has ended.

- *Long term:* If you have breathing difficulties like asthma, changes to your breathing can make it difficult to get enough oxygen. Breathing hard can also cause you to hyperventilate.

HEART

- *Short term:* Your heart pumps blood around your body at a faster rate. The blood vessels around the heart dilate to allow more blood to travel to your muscles. This raises your blood pressure.

- *Long term:* You can be left with a consistently raised heartbeat and high blood pressure. This together with stress hormones can increase your chances of a heart attack or stroke. It can even affect your cholesterol levels.

MUSCLES

- *Short term:* Muscles tense up, allowing your body to spring into action, but will relax straight afterwards.

- *Long term:* If your muscles are constantly tense it will affect other muscles, tendons, and joints and may lead to injuries. It can also cause tension headaches and migraines.

DIGESTION

- *Short term:* You might feel nauseous or even vomit. You can have short-term diarrhoea or constipation.

- *Long term:* Can lead to chronic changes in your digestion or eating habits. Your ability to absorb nutrients will be compromised. You may develop acid reflux.

HORMONES

- *Short term:* Stress hormones and increased blood sugar give your body more energy.

- *Long term:* If you don't reabsorb the extra blood sugar then you could develop diabetes. Cortisol can lead to thyroid problems and weight gain.

REPRODUCTIVE SYSTEMS

- *Short term:* Blood supply will be directed temporarily away from the reproductive organs.

- *Long term:* Can affect production of sperm and testosterone in men. Can also cause erectile disfunction. In women it can worsen or trigger menopause and change the menstrual cycle. In both cases, it can decrease libido.

IMMUNE SYSTEM

- *Short term:* The immune system is temporarily decreased.

- *Long term:* More vulnerable to infection and illnesses. Recovery time is longer.

FIG. 18.2

HOW STRESS AND ANXIETY AFFECT YOUR BODY

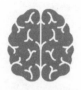

Poor concentration,
makes you more irritable,
and gives you brain fog

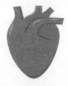

Raised cholesterol levels
and blood pressure

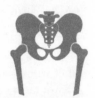

Increased inflammation and
tension, leading to aches
and tightness in your muscles

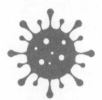

Decreased immunity
and longer recovery times

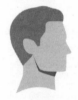

Hair loss, weakened nails,
and can contribute to
dry skin and acne which
can take longer to heal

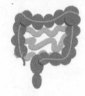

Affects the absorption of
nutrients by the body and can
lead to constipation, diarrhoea,
bloating, and indigestion

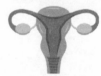

Decreased sex drive and
hormone production,
and increased PMS symptoms

WHAT IS ANXIETY?

Anxiety is also part of the body's response when in 'fight or flight' mode. It is a natural response that is designed to keep us safe. It is completely normal to feel nervous or a bit anxious before a big event or when we might miss our bus. It encourages us to be on high alert, sharpens our thinking, and makes us poised for action.

Stress and anxiety often appear to be interchangeable, but there is a difference between the two. Generally speaking, stress is a reaction to an outside factor, whereas anxiety is the internal response to stress. If we go back to our 4.30 p.m. deadline, this would be considered a source of stress as it is external. However, we might react to it in very different ways. One person might sail through the task, high on the feeling of productivity that their stress response has produced. The other will be equally capable of producing exceptional work, but at the same time they will be suffering from anxiety about the task. They'll worry that they will make a mistake, be uneasy about why they were given the task, and be fearful of missing the deadline. Negative anxious thoughts are the internal reaction to the external source of stress.

In short, stress is the physical and mental demands placed on us; anxiety is when we react to them with high levels of fear, worry, or unease.

Another difference between stress and anxiety is how long they last for. The stress response tends to melt away once the source of stress passes (unless there are repeated sources of stress, such as more deadlines or missed credit card payments). Anxiety has the potential to linger even when the original source of stress has disappeared. Normal levels of anxiety should pass once the stressful event is concluded, but for people with anxiety conditions it won't, and they remain in that heightened, alert state.

Like the stress response, short-term anxiety also has a physical effect on our body. It raises our heartbeat and blood pressure, and we may sweat more. It can also affect our thinking patterns and we might become more focused. However, if we have long-term anxiety, we might suffer from overthinking, ruminate on past events, worry constantly, or even suffer from memory loss (see Figure 18.3). This in turn can affect all areas of our life. We might have difficulty sleeping, avoid certain situations, have a short temper, or require constant reassurance.

FIG. 18.3
HOW TO RECOGNIZE ANXIETY IN YOURSELF AND OTHERS

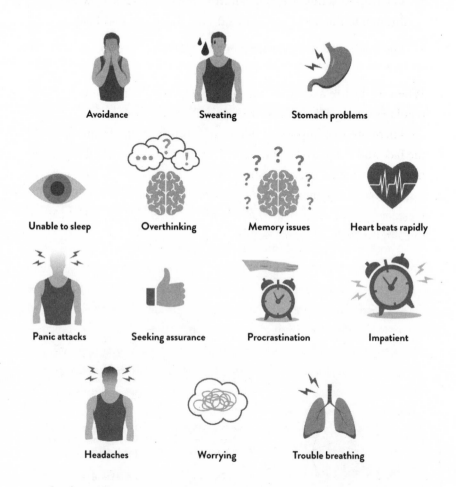

Avoidance   Sweating   Stomach problems

Unable to sleep   Overthinking   Memory issues   Heart beats rapidly

Panic attacks   Seeking assurance   Procrastination   Impatient

Headaches   Worrying   Trouble breathing

HOW I TREAT STRESS AND ANXIETY THROUGH THERAPY

Treatment from a therapist can encourage a balance between the two systems that moderate our stress response, and can help with both the acute and chronic effects of stress and anxiety. Tension is often held in the body, which can be released through massage and dry needling. Muscles that commonly hold tension from stress and anxiety are:

- The suboccipital muscles at the back of the head

- The strong masseter muscle around the jaw

- The trapezius muscles that run from under the skull, down through to the neck, and across the shoulder and mid-back.

- The intercostal muscles between the ribs

When we feel relaxed our 'rest and digest' system takes over, which regulates our mood and improves sleep and digestion.

There are two important nerves that run from the brain, through the face and down to the abdomen. Together they are called the vagus nerve. The vagus nerve is the longest cranial nerve in the body, is responsible for helping with the 'rest and digest' response, and sends messages from the brain to our organs (see Figure 18.4), thus helping to calm the 'fight or flight' response.

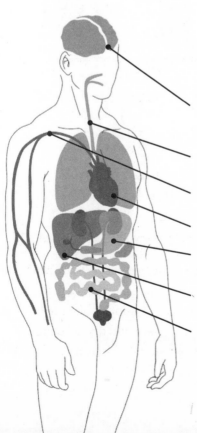

FIG. 18.4
HOW THE VAGUS NERVE AFFECTS
ORGAN SYSTEMS

Helps keep anxiety and depression at bay. Opposes the sympathetic response to stress.

Taste information is sent via three cranial nerves, one of which is the vagus nerve. The vagus nerve is needed for the gag reflex, swallowing and coughing.

Decreases vascular tone, lowering blood pressure.

Decreases heart rate and vascular tone.

Increases gastric juices, gut motility and stomach acidity.

Regulates insulin secretion and glucose homeostasis in the liver.

Suppresses inflammation via the cholinergic anti-inflammatory pathway.

There are three points in the ear that are acupressure points that can treat the vagus nerve. This can be done by a skilled therapist, or you could try it at home. Begin by massaging the three points in Figure 18.5 with the tip of your finger, for one minute each. Finish off by pinching the outer cartilage of the ear. After doing this, take a minute to check if your breathing is steadier and if you are feeling more relaxed.

I also treat my vagus nerve by humming or singing. This is because the nerve is linked to the vocal chords and the muscles surrounding the throat. I also do cold exposure through taking ice baths and cold showers, but even something as simple as splashing your face with cold water can be effective in regulating your stress.

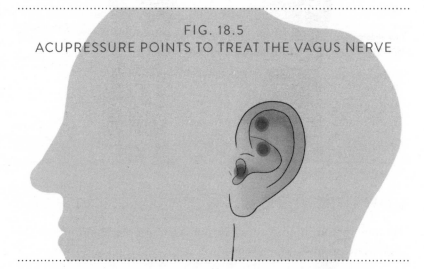

FIG. 18.5
ACUPRESSURE POINTS TO TREAT THE VAGUS NERVE

One thing that I regularly teach my clients is how to breathe through their abdomen rather than just their chest. People who carry visible signs of stress and anxiety in their bodies often have rounded shoulders or their shoulders are raised towards their ears. These postures can also affect how we breathe and if we can change this our body begins to uncurl and relax. Through 'belly breathing' we naturally lower our heartbeat, which in turn helps to reduce feelings of stress or anxiety. An experienced osteopath or therapist can help you learn deep breathing exercises with the aim of releasing tension in the diaphragm, chest, and neck (see Figure 18.6).

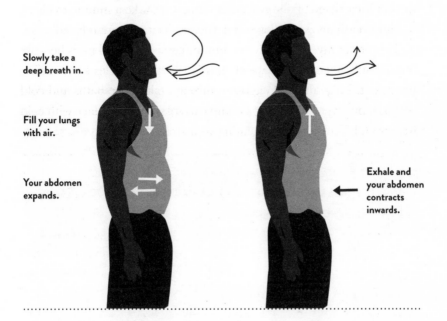

FIG 18.6
BREATHING THROUGH YOUR ABDOMEN

Slowly take a
deep breath in.

Fill your lungs
with air.

Your abdomen
expands.

Exhale and
your abdomen
contracts
inwards.

HOW I TREAT STRESS AND ANXIETY AT HOME

Treatment from both a therapist and at home can help relieve the symptoms of stress and anxiety and encourage our 'rest and digest' mode to restore balance. But when it comes to chronic stress or anxiety, often the only way to tackle this is through a more long-term lifestyle change. This is what happened to me when I finished the 2016 Olympics and went back into private practice. I was completely burnt out from the stress of the previous years and threw myself back into seeing at least ten patients a day in my private practice, as well as juggling the responsibilities of home life.

I see this in so many of my patients. They're in their forties, fifties, and sixties and just holding out for retirement. They're burnt out, stressed out, and their bodies are not functioning properly. They tell me that once they earn a certain amount of money or achieve a particular promotion, they'll think about cutting back. They view their retirement as a golden time when they will have saved enough to live the way they have always dreamed of. I treat them, patch them up, and encourage them to look after themselves at home, but often they don't because they are too busy and tired.

I have patients who I have treated for ten years or more, so I get to see what happens when their retirement finally comes around. They are usually in chronic pain, battling with various conditions and illnesses. They might have diabetes, heart disease, or cancer. Arthritis might have crept into their bodies, refusing to let go. When they dreamed about their retirement, they had imagined themselves being healthy and fit, able to do anything they wanted. Instead, their bodies are exhausted and, sadly, irreversible damage has often been done.

I understand that a lifestyle change cannot be achieved overnight and for some people it feels unattainable, or a source of stress in itself. Therefore, the following chapters are about what we can do in our day-to-day lives to break those cycles of stress and anxiety, recognize the messages our bodies are sending us, and keep our bodies supple to prevent injuries and other conditions.

But before I do that, I'd like to share my first tips on what helps me regulate my stress response at home and brings me back to that balanced, calm state. Maybe you will find something that you can put into practice in your own life.

An often unacknowledged part of being a good therapist is being a good listener. My clients often tell me what is on their mind as I treat them, and I feel privileged to be someone who they trust. This ability to share our thoughts also crosses over into treating stress and anxiety at home. I honestly believe that what helps me balance my long working hours with the other responsibilities in my life is a strong network of people who I regularly speak to. I am blessed to have several like-minded people who I speak to every week. They celebrate my wins with me and commiserate on my losses, and I trust their advice. This human interaction is what stabilizes me, calms me, and allows my body to remain in balance.

MY TOP TIPS FOR REDUCING STRESS AND ANXIETY:

- Find like-minded people who you can talk to regularly.

- Go outside by yourself and take a few minutes to connect with nature.

When I was young and everything was getting on top of me, my mum told me to have a glass of water, go outside, look at the natural world, and take a deep breath. At the time I thought she had missed the mark by a long way. Now that I'm in my thirties, I find myself outside most mornings staring up at the sky. I go outside in the evenings too, so I can see the stars. Perhaps you're reading this and thinking I'm missing the mark, but just try it. Take yourself outside. Don't speak, don't try to film it, or share it with a friend – just look up and take a few deep breaths. Realize how small you are in comparison to everything else out there. It provides perspective, allowing you to step away from yourself for just a few moments – a chance for your overstimulated body to reset.

Because that's what tackling our response to stress and anxiety is all about – giving our body a chance to reset – and there is more about this in Chapter 19.

CHAPTER 19

The 360° approach:

SPACE

W e've managed to heal ourselves and no longer have a lingering pain in our back or knee. But why do we still have twinges, feel sluggish in the morning, and are wide awake by bedtime? These are all pre-pain messages from our body that we are not looking after it properly. Until we have a self-care programme that resets our body's stress levels and prevents injuries and other health conditions, we are in limbo rather than in prevention mode. We want to be in an optimal state of health where we are energized but also calm; focused but also relaxed.

One of the reasons I stand out at what I do is that I don't just think about the problem that is presented to me and how to treat it. Instead, I look at a client's lifestyle as a whole. I look at the fine detail. I don't want to just fix the problem in the short term; I want to make sure it doesn't come back. The client needs to be aware of how they got into this position and then it's up to them to decide if they want to change those contributing factors.

People need to live in the now. They need to take care of themselves right now, not in ten, twenty, or thirty years' time, because it might be too late by then. You owe that to yourself, and you will be better at the things that are important to you if you do. It's not just about dealing

" People need to live in the now.
They need to take care of
themselves before it's too late. "

with pain; it's about looking at the clues that have led you to this place, and then setting rituals that are realistic. I want people to feel good about themselves, and to start this process you need to listen to the clues that your body is giving you.

Think about your answers to the following questions:

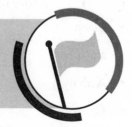

- When you woke up this morning, did your body feel stiff?
- Was it hard to walk around?
- Do you find it difficult getting up from a chair?
- Are you out of breath by the time you get to the top of the stairs?
- Do you constantly reach for your neck and shoulders and rub them without even noticing?
- Do you have general aches across your body?
- Do you feel tired all the time?
- Is it difficult to keep up with your children?
- Are you gaining weight around your stomach?
- Do you find it difficult to fall asleep?
- Has your libido reduced?
- Are your nails brittle?
- Are you having skin outbreaks, such as spots?

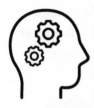 These are just some messages our body can send us and if you're receiving them, it's time to turn into your own detective. We do this by giving ourselves **SPACE** and checking in on all areas of our wellbeing, where SPACE relates to the following areas in our lives.

- **S**leep
- **P**osture
- **A**ctivity
- **C**alm
- **E**nergy

The following sections look at the above in more detail.

SLEEP

Sleep is one of those things we cannot go without. Like water and food, if you don't sleep, your systems will eventually shut down. Nowadays, we often treat sleep as a weakness. Have you ever heard a colleague mention that they never sleep more than five hours a night? That they work regular twelve-hour days? You might get a twinge of self-doubt or wish you could do something similar. We shouldn't be impressed, because internally their body is struggling to function. They will age faster, have a weakened immune system, be less interested in sex, store more fat, and be at a higher risk of heart disease and diabetes (see Figure 19.1). Doesn't have the same ring to it now, does it?

Sleep is the ultimate recharger and chance to reset after a stress response. It also helps to heal and repair our bodies. The best place to start is with eight hours sleep, but some people will need slightly more and others less. The minimum you should be having is six hours a night and it's likely that your body will need more than this. After one night of little or no sleep, we will be tired and often short-tempered. If this rolls on for many days, weeks, or months it will affect our general health and mood. We won't be able to think as clearly, and our immune system will become compromised. If you can, you could try topping up your sleep with naps during the day, but it's better to have it all in one go at night.

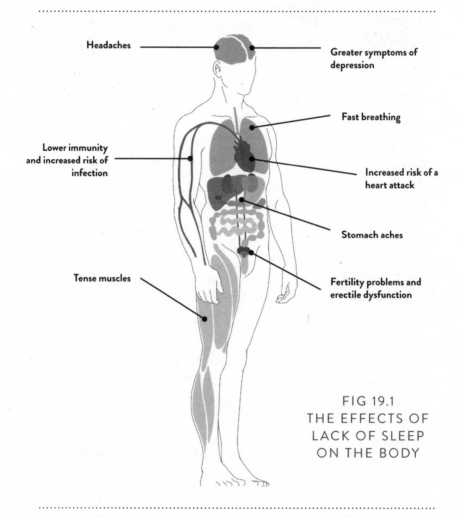

FIG 19.1
THE EFFECTS OF
LACK OF SLEEP
ON THE BODY

This is because the quality of our sleep is also important. If we are constantly waking up, then we can't access the deep sleep, where the body repairs, nor the later REM sleep, which aids our mental processes. We cycle through the four stages of sleep throughout the night and if we are woken up, the cycle must restart and there is less balance between them (see Figure 19.2). We tend to have more deep

FIG. 19.2
THE FOUR STAGES OF SLEEP

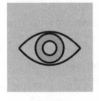

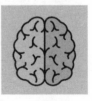

Awake   **Light sleep**   **Deep sleep**   **REM sleep**

sleep in the first hours and more REM in the later ones. Research shows that we get more deep sleep before midnight and therefore eight hours of sleep that includes time before midnight is better than eight hours after midnight.

Ways that we can help ourselves to have more quality sleep and fall asleep earlier are:

- Wearing a sleep mask

- Blacking out our bedroom

- Leaving our phone in another room

- Limiting TV before bed

- Limiting the use of electronics such as laptops, iPads, and Kindles

- Using natural sleep supplements

In the last few years, I have been treating most of my clients in their homes. This means that I can assess how they sit on their sofa or at the dinner table, their sleeping position and how many pillows they use during the night. I'm always asked what the best type of mattress and pillows are. My advice is that it isn't as simple as just mattresses and pillows. What's really important is our sleeping position (see Figure 19.3), and whether it is right for any of the medical conditions we might have. The position in which we sleep can affect our blood flow, oxygen supply, and hormone production. Consequently, it can also affect our ability to heal, our digestion, and blood pressure.

The older you get, the more important your sleeping position is. In an ideal world, a therapist will assess how you sleep and whether this is aiding or even causing any health conditions that you have. If this is outside of your budget, then there are a few tips below on how you could adapt your sleeping position to the messages your body is sending.

FIG. 19.3
MOST POPULAR SLEEPING POSITIONS

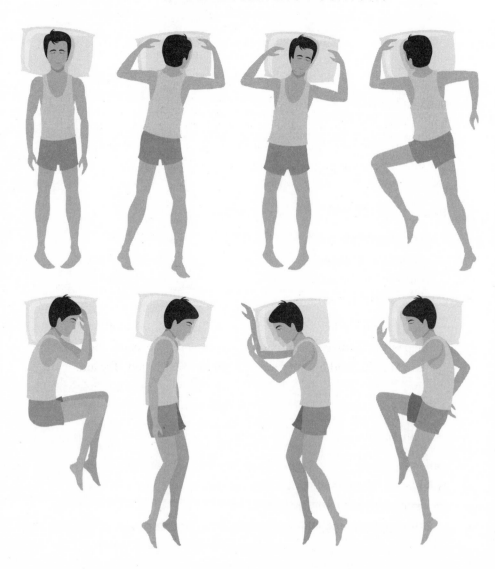

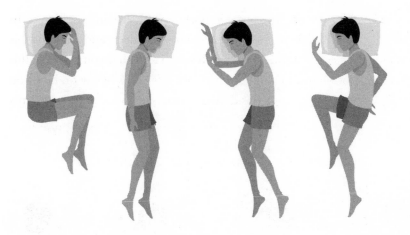

SIDE-SLEEPING

Most of us sleep on our sides, sometimes curled up as we would have been before we were born. I am a side sleeper and try to sleep on my left side. There are pros and cons of side-sleeping:

Pros

- Side-sleeping is good for stopping snoring as it helps improve our breathing through clearer airways.

- Sleeping on the left side can help with digestive issues, such as acid reflux and heartburn.

- Sleeping in the foetal position can help with lower-back pain, particularly if you place a pillow between your knees.

- It is the recommended sleeping position for the later trimesters of pregnancy.

Cons

- Sleeping on your right side can increase issues, such as acid reflux and heartburn.

- Side-sleeping can cause pins and needles or numbness in your hands because the blood flow is disrupted. Try and move your shoulder slightly forward to alleviate this.

- It's not very good for weak shoulders.

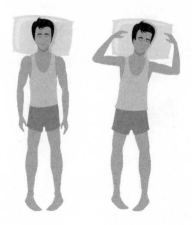

BACK IS BEST

In general terms, it is thought that sleeping on our back is the best position, but this depends on the health conditions you have.

Pros

- Sleeping on your back is good for the spine as it allows all the nutrients to flow freely into your discs overnight.

- It is also beneficial for your hips and knees.

- It's good for digestion.

- Reduces the risk of acid reflux.

Cons

- It can sometimes feel uncomfortable with lower-back pain. One way to alleviate this it to place a pillow underneath your knees as this takes the pressure off your lower spine.

- It can sometimes feel uncomfortable for neck pain.

- There is a greater likelihood of snoring and sleep apnoea in this position.

- Sleeping on your back is not recommended for women in their third trimester of pregnancy.

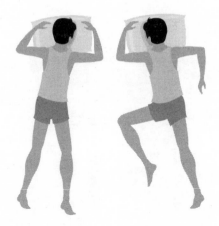

FRONT DOWN

Sleeping on your front is generally thought of as the worst position to sleep, but some negatives can be reduced with a few simple adjustments.

Pros

- It's the best position to stop snoring and sleep apnoea.

- If you sleep face-down, rather than turning your head to the side, it keeps your upper airways clear and open.

Cons

- This can be the most damaging position for your neck as one side of the neck muscles can lengthen, while the other shortens. There is also the risk of your neck joints locking during the night.

- It can also put strain on your spine, which can put strain on your muscles, tendons, and joints.

If you can't change position, then it's better to have one of your knees lifted to the side and keep your arms raised rather than by your side. There will also be a lot of pressure on your spine if you have high pillows in this position, so it is better to have a lower pillow (see Figure 19.4). You can also place a flat pillow underneath your stomach to take the pressure off your lower back.

FIG. 19.4
RIGHT PILLOW POSITION

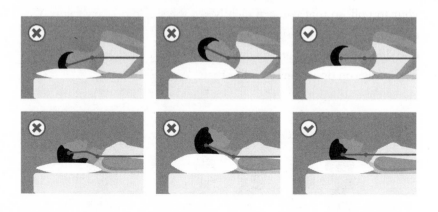

Pillows are very important as we need to keep our spine as straight as possible during the night. For a similar reason, mattresses shouldn't be too soft, or we sink into them and our spine curves. Over the years, I have noticed a pattern with patients who get neck, shoulder, and lower-back pain. This often happens because they have slept on a sofa, in a friend's spare room, or at a hotel where they didn't have the right pillow, or the bed was too soft. I always recommend that my clients take their own pillows or mattress toppers with them if they can. When I was a therapist for the Great Britain team, we did this with nearly sixty track and field athletes so we could prevent avoidable injuries. Mattress toppers are useful because they can adjust the surface of a bed, so it is more suited to your sleeping position, without the need to buy a new mattress.

POSTURE

Whenever I meet someone new, even if they're not a client, I always end up assessing their posture. It's second nature now and tells me what potential health problems they might have. It comes from when I was at university and we would spend hours studying another student's posture from the front, back, and side. We had to sketch how they stood and note down any asymmetries or abnormalities.

You can check your own posture by using a camera stand, or asking someone to take a picture of your side, back, and front, preferably with your top off, so that you can clearly see the shape of your spine. You should also check whether your shoulders are level. It is common for one side to be lower than the other and this is often caused by carrying heavy bags on one shoulder (see Figure 19.5).

FIG. 19.5
WHICH POSTURE ARE YOU?

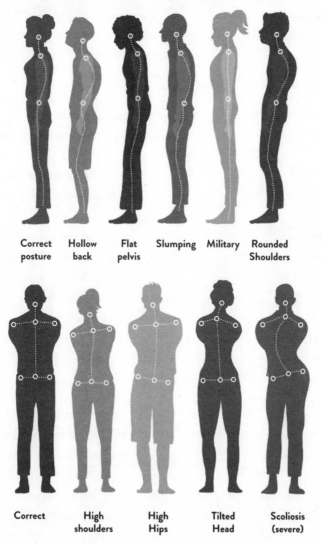

| Correct posture | Hollow back | Flat pelvis | Slumping | Military | Rounded Shoulders |

| Correct | High shoulders | High Hips | Tilted Head | Scoliosis (severe) |

We live in a time when we need advice on our posture as we often don't do the things our body needs, or we force it into unnatural positions for long periods of time. Our posture can be affected by the demands of our job – a post office worker will have different physical demands to a plumber. Other lifestyle factors are if we play sport in our spare time, or if we don't feel very confident, as we might try and shrink ourselves when out in public.

There are many internal factors that can affect our posture as well. It might be that scoliosis in part of the spine is causing it to curve to the side. We might have one leg slightly longer than the other that shifts our weight onto the other one (see Figure 19.6), or an extra rib or section of the spine, which might put added pressure on other internal structures.

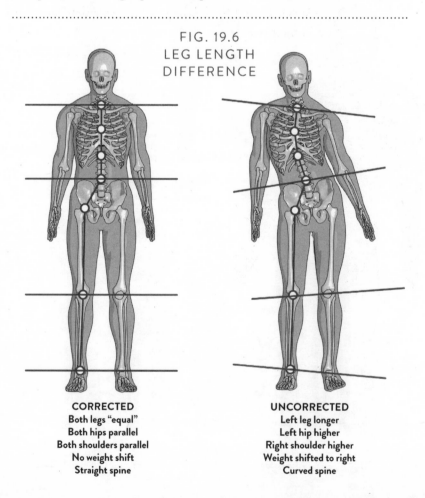

FIG. 19.6
LEG LENGTH
DIFFERENCE

CORRECTED
Both legs "equal"
Both hips parallel
Both shoulders parallel
No weight shift
Straight spine

UNCORRECTED
Left leg longer
Left hip higher
Right shoulder higher
Weight shifted to right
Curved spine

Our age also plays a huge part as our posture changes as we grow into adulthood and also during pregnancy. There is also the impact of pain to consider, where we adapt our posture into a protective one so we don't aggravate it. There can also be illnesses or diseases that affect our joints and bones, such as arthritis. When considering what might be altering our posture, we really do need to look at every aspect of our lives.

What's so great about good posture? The main things are that it takes less energy to maintain, it helps us breathe better and, most importantly, it doesn't impact on other areas of our body. Once we start adjusting our postures, other parts become strained and overloaded, causing a ripple effect of damage. This is called an 'antalgic posture' (see Figure 19.7), and is more common than you would expect. I often see it when people have damaged discs in their back.

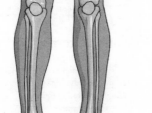

FIG. 19.7
ANTALGIC POSTURE

Antalgic posture happens when the person leans to one side to avoid pain on the opposite side.

Prolonged antalgic posture can cause muscle imbalances, which could lead to other issues.

The two most common abnormal postures that I see are abnormal kyphosis or lordosis and these are the ones you are most likely to notice if you have taken photos of your posture.

HYPER-KYPHOSIS

This is when the curve in the mid-back is exaggerated (see Figure 19.8). Along with this curvature of the spine, the person's shoulders are normally rounded and their head tilts forward. You will most clearly be able to see this in a side view of yourself.

The exaggerated round curve is commonly in the mid-back, rather than the neck or lower back. There are several reasons why this can happen, but it is often because of poor posture (carrying heavy bags, slouching, hunching over a desk or steering wheel) and

FIG. 19.8
HYPER-KYPHOSIS OF THE SPINE

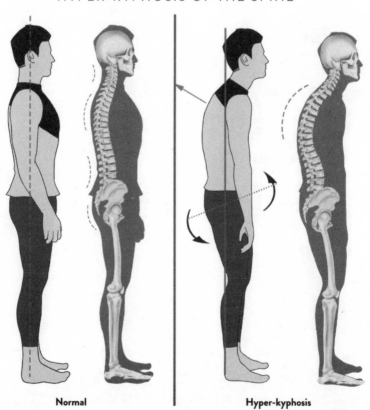

Normal   Hyper-kyphosis

is more noticeable in older people. It can be symptomless, but will normally cause muscle aches and tenderness. Pain from this condition will normally be centred around the shoulders and neck. The way to offset this condition is to use regular exercises to open up your chest, foam roller your mid-back, and practise moving your shoulder blades together. There will be more about this in Chapter 20.

HYPER-LORDOSIS

The lower back curves naturally, but if it is exaggerated, it is called hyper-lordosis (see Figure 19.9). This will also be visible from a side view of your body. It can happen in the neck as well, but is more common in the lower back. It will cause muscle pain and sometimes stiffness in the back.

FIG. 19.9
HYPER-LORDOSIS OF THE SPINE

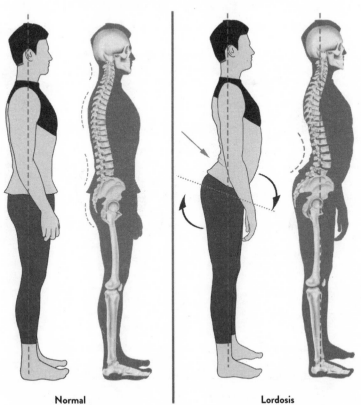

Normal   Lordosis

It is thought that standing or sitting for long periods of time partly contribute to this condition. Therefore, these two activities should be broken up throughout the day with some of the exercises in Chapter 20. It has also been linked to sleeping on the stomach, so try to change your sleeping position if you can.

There are so many subtle ways that we adjust our postures from a young age and these changes form into habits. They spread across our homes and workspaces: the way we clean the dishes, sit on the sofa or sit at our desk, and how we sleep. In the last few decades, hand-held devices have been introduced into our lives and they have had an overwhelming impact on our posture. When we use an iPad, phone, or laptop we tend to look down at them and this position is unhealthy for the spine in the long term. But if we are aware of this, we can begin to take steps to limit their impact, by doing some of the following:

- Check your posture throughout the day with either a mirror or camera, or ask someone else to check it for you

- Limit your time on your phone or devices if you can

- Get a hands-free kit for your phone so you can move about freely when on calls

- Try using voice texting (if your phone has that feature) because it doesn't require you to look down as much

- Do stretches and exercises throughout the day to maintain posture (Chapter 20 will cover these)

- Position your devices so they are at eye level

- Have regular breaks from sitting down

TIPS FOR SITTING AT A DESK

- Keep your back straight

- Don't roll your shoulders inwards or too far backwards

- Keep your feet flat on the ground

- Place your screen so it is directly in front of your eye line

- Your knees should be bent at a 90-degree angle

- Your elbows should be close to your sides and bent between 90 and 120 degrees

- Consider switching your chair for an exercise ball throughout the day for half an hour

- Take regular breaks to walk around your work area

- Break up periods of being seated with some of the exercises in Chapter 20

- Consider investing in an ergonomic chair if you have back pain

TIPS FOR STANDING

- Place your feet shoulder-width apart

- Spread your weight evenly between both legs

- Let your arms relax by your sides

- Look straight ahead when you can

- Be aware of your shoulders rolling in and try to correct them

- Try to stand up tall, rather than slouch

- If you can, wear compression socks

LYING IN BED (RATHER THAN SLEEPING)

- Don't lie on your back with several pillows under your head as this tips your neck forward. Instead, build up several pillows to support your back

- Place a pillow under your knees to take pressure away from your lower back

- If you are lying on your side, curl your legs up in the foetal position and try not to put all your weight through your shoulder. Instead, move it slightly forwards.

LIFTING

- When carrying a heavy load, pull it in towards your body rather than holding it out in front of you.

- When picking something up from the ground, keep your spine straight rather than looking down at the object you are lifting. Bend at your knees rather than your hips and engage your core muscles. Use your leg muscles to lift rather than your back.

DRIVING

- Sit upright

- Your seat should accommodate the curve in your lower back (see Figure 19.10)

- If you are driving for long periods, then try some of the gentle stretches in Chapter 20

FIG. 19.10
CORRECT DRIVING POSITION

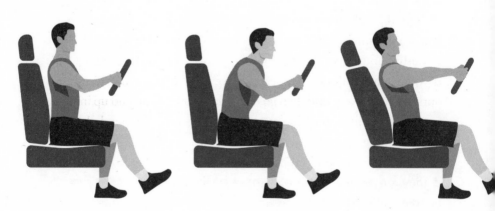

Correct   Incorrect   Incorrect

ACTIVE

We are designed to move throughout the day and once we stop doing this, and responding to what our body needs, other medical conditions begin to set in. Our jobs often require us to stay in one place for hours at a time. This is why I have devised exercises in Chapter 20, whereby you can multitask between the demands of your day and using gentle stretches to counteract them. Chapter 20 covers all the stretches and exercises that your body needs to keep you active. We also don't have to devote as much time to exercise if we try to keep our bodies moving throughout the day.

The benefits of activity are huge. Studies show that if we exercise regularly, it can help prevent health conditions such as cancer, heart conditions, strokes, osteoarthritis, diabetes, dementia, and depression. There are even research studies that show that being active can reduce the chance of you developing a major health condition by up to 50 per cent. If you already have a health condition, then being active can also help manage it.

Activity also helps regulate our mood as we are answering a request from our body. It is natural for our body to expect to exercise every day. It will crave this and reward us with a release of endorphins when we respond to it.

The flip side from too little activity is too much intense activity. It is very common that we can go from sitting down for eight hours to pushing ourselves during a two-hour workout in the evening. This is when many injuries happen. Or we have a manual job, exhaust ourselves every day, and then go on to play football and end up injuring ourselves. If this is something you do, then you should spend plenty of time warming up and cooling down to prepare your body for intensive exercise. You should also be alert to any new twinges in your body – if they are getting worse or happen in the same area of your body between different exercise sessions then it's a sign that something isn't quite right and needs further investigation.

There are lots of people who look incredibly healthy and fit on the outside, but internally their bodies are suffering from the stress of being constantly overworked. They're always on the go, never giving their body the chance to wind down into that balanced neutral state. In its extreme form, this can cause heart conditions. I know of several middle-aged people who have exercised hard, running marathons or doing Iron Mans, and then had a stroke or heart attack. Our bodies need time to rest and time to heal between exercise sessions. If we don't give them this opportunity, then we are piling stressor on top of stressor and eventually there will be a negative result. If this sounds like you, then the next section is very important.

CALM

In Chapter 18 I talked about the two contrasting states that need to be balanced, our 'fight and flight' and 'rest and digest'. If we are constantly in 'fight or flight' mode, and don't allow our bodies to come down from this heightened state, then many of our essential systems cannot function properly.

To enter a state of calm, we should start by removing ourselves from those outside stress factors for a short time: that is, the emails, the work calls, the demands placed on us by others. If we can just put aside even ten minutes without those outside stressors, then it is a good start and we will hopefully allow our 'rest and digest' mode to calm us. It also gives us a chance to take a step back from what was previously absorbing our attention and gain some perspective on it. We might even try and make more time for ourselves as a result.

> "START BY REMOVING OURSELVES FROM OUTSIDE STRESS FACTORS."

Often when we take ourselves away from these outside stressors, we can't leave that heightened state. We are so switched on that we cannot come down and instead spend our ten minutes worrying about what is coming next, or whether we did something correctly. There are several ways of dealing with this. I like to tackle it by doing something that focuses my attention on the present – often I am focused on the future or pulled back into the past. It's about finding something that works for you to bring you back to this very moment. Some people find meditation or mindfulness helps, or practising gratitude; others might use their breathing, gentle exercise such as yoga, or journaling. Try all these things, as what is relaxing for one person might not work for another. There is no right or wrong answer, it just has to hold you in the present so you are not ruminating on the past or planning for the future.

The following are a couple of things that work best for me.

SAUNAS

I am a huge fan of saunas. The heat is very relaxing while also placing beneficial stress on the body that causes the following to happen:

- Skin temperature rises, which increases the circulation to the skin

- Heart rate increases

- Sweating increases

I've had some of my best ideas in a sauna as the heat forces me to stay in the present and my mind can access its creative side. Studies also show that there are several possible health benefits from saunas including: reducing stress and anxiety, lowering blood pressure, increasing circulation, aiding respiratory issues (I've found my breathing has deepened since using saunas), speeding up the recovery of overworked muscles, and improving sleep. There is even a study from Finland with a small test group that shows that regular saunas might improve life expectancy. If you do decide to give saunas a go, then you should drink plenty of water before and afterwards and don't stay in for more than twenty minutes.

> "I'VE HAD SOME OF MY BEST IDEAS IN A SAUNA."

WALKS

One of the most stressful times of my life was when I was abroad working with the Olympic team. I lived and breathed my work, never switching off or taking time to look after myself. I woke up in the morning and considered what I could do to help the athletes and thought about this all the way through the day until I fell into bed completely exhausted.

The only way I could get myself out of this cycle was to take myself off for a walk. There was no direction or purpose to it, it was just me gently moving my body while my brain got to see different sights that calmed and soothed it. I still use this now, even if I only have time for a short walk around my garden between calls. It helps me relax for a few minutes and eases me into a calmer place for the rest of the day.

There are so many people I know who think that they are being selfish if they take this time for themselves. The demands of their work or home life, or both, pull them in every direction and they always end up coming last. The way I see it is if you want to be better at your passion, or your job, or looking after other people, then you have to take time for yourself. It isn't selfish to be in the best condition to meet the demands placed on you. You should never feel guilty for wanting to look after yourself as well as everyone else you love.

> "SO MANY PEOPLE THINK THEY ARE SELFISH IF THEY TAKE TIME FOR THEMSELVES."

ENERGY

Lack of energy is another sign from your body that it isn't getting what it needs. If you don't have the energy to complete everything that is needed during the day or you are absolutely exhausted by the end of it, these are both clear signs that things aren't right. We need to think about whether our energy battery is green, orange, or red. Besides the classic symptom of tiredness, a lack of energy may also show itself as being unable to think clearly, having difficulty concentrating, or feeling unmotivated. First, you should check with a doctor that there isn't a medical condition such as a thyroid problem, hormonal imbalance, low blood sugar, or sleep apnoea that is causing your fatigue. If this isn't the case, then you might need to look at what is going into your body and what you are expelling. If these things don't weigh up, they need to be adjusted.

WE NEED TO FIRSTLY LOOK AT WHAT IS GOING INTO US:

- Are you eating enough nutritious food? Have an honest, hard look at what you are eating. Are you getting the right balance of food types in your diet? If you aren't, then there is a lot of information on the internet to help you improve this, or you could book an appointment with a nutritionist.

- Are you drinking enough water? This is a very common problem and being dehydrated can lead to low energy and fatigue. How much water we need to drink varies between each individual, but a general aim is to drink six to eight glasses of water a day, which is about 1.2 to 1.5 litres.

- Are you getting enough sleep? There is more about sleep above (see pages 347–54), but if we aren't getting the sleep that our body needs, then we will not have enough energy the following day.

WE NEED TO THEN CONSIDER WHAT WE ARE EXPENDING OUR ENERGY ON:

- Are you doing too much? Have a think about whether you are always racing from one place to the next. You might not feel negative stress from these things, but even constant positive stress is detrimental to your body.

- Are you allowing yourself to rest at regular intervals, or not? Does your body rarely get the chance to allow the 'rest and digest' response to calm you and enable your body to focus on all the background functions that we often ignore.

- Are you expending all your energy on other people? This can have both a mental and physical effect. When I was a therapist in private practice, I found that my energy was given to all my patients through my constant interactions, and trying to heal and empathize with them. I was giving all my energy to everyone else and after ten years of this, it was no longer sustainable. I had to cut back on the number of patients I saw. This can also occur in our personal lives with friends, partners and people we regularly speak to who we expend so much energy caring for, listening to, advising, supporting, and propping up. Years slip by and we are still giving everything to them, and so we have to ask ourselves if they are giving something back.

- Are we expending all our energy on our work? If so, this leaves little time to perform the basic tasks that you need to keep your own body balanced. We need to have a chance to rest so our body can repair itself. We also need to feed it properly, keep it active, clean, and cared for. If we don't have time for these simple, essential tasks then our lives are out of balance.

Take a look at the two sides to your energy and, if you can, try to increase the beneficial things that are going into your body and consider reducing what you are expending your precious energy on.

There are also two methods that I use to quickly raise my energy levels when needed:

ICE BATHS

These are something that I recommend to 95 per cent of my clients. I have an ice bath and cold shower every day and I can honestly say that it has changed my mind and body. It makes me feel incredibly focused and it is during an ice bath that I have some of my most creative ideas. I find that this blast of cold helps with muscle soreness, speeds up my metabolism, reduces inflammation, and improves my energy levels.

You can build up to a full ice bath by starting off with having a cold shower for a few seconds, but I would recommend a full ice bath to get all the benefits. You shouldn't stay in longer than fifteen minutes; and even a few seconds are beneficial. Build up to longer times in an ice bath and always check with your doctor if you're concerned about whether it is suitable for you to do. If you don't have a bath at home, then have ice-cold showers as these will help produce the same effect.

SURROUND YOURSELF WITH POSITIVE PEOPLE

This is crucial when it comes to energy. A conversation with someone who you know will always have something positive or inspiring to say can lift you up in just a few minutes. If you spend your time with positive, energetic people you can't help but absorb it.

SPACE (**S**leep, **P**osture, **A**ctivity, **C**alm and **E**nergy) is what we should bear in mind when trying to ensure our general wellbeing. Take the time to run through these five things whenever something doesn't feel quite right within yourself. The aim is to restore all these areas so that you feel energized and balanced, and to help prevent future illnesses and medical conditions.

CHAPTER 20

Activity

If we don't include activity in our daily lives, we become part of the myth that pain naturally increases as we age. Pain in our old age is often preventable. It usually occurs because we haven't kept our joints, muscles, tendons, and ligaments supple during our younger years. But it doesn't have to be this way. If we start incorporating gentle exercises and stretches into our daily routine and add some cardio, then we are giving ourselves a much better chance to continue doing the things we love right into our old age.

People are living longer. In the period 2018–2020, the median age for life expectancy was 82.3 for men and 85.8 for women. This means we need to start forging good habits now to ensure we keep as much function as we get older. I've had clients in their nineties who can still hold a squat because they have always squatted while eating. Their bodies are perfectly tuned to this position, so they keep on doing it. Of course, there will be some injuries and medical conditions that we can't do anything to prevent, but what I'm talking about is the gradual decrease in movement that comes with a body that isn't kept supple.

Ask yourself, do you want to be able to keep up with the demands of your job completely pain-free or do you want to continue having nagging aches in your back and neck that increase over the years,

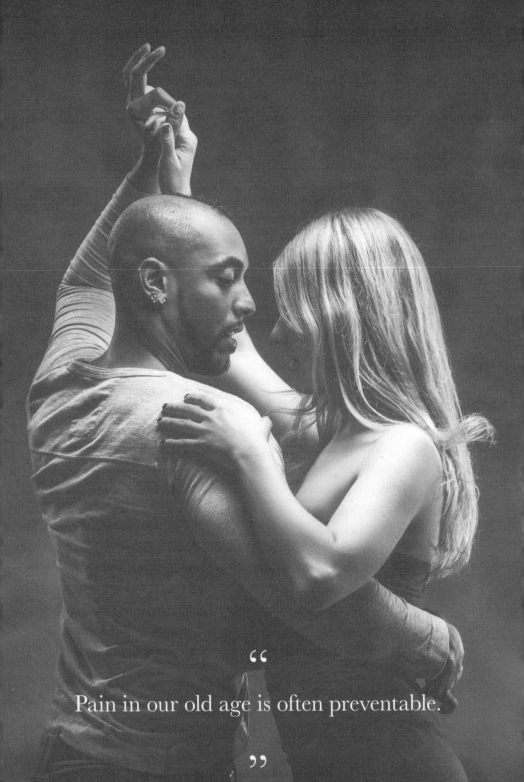

“
Pain in our old age is often preventable.
”

eventually limiting the work you can do? Do you want to be someone who can keep up with your children as they grow into energetic teenagers, or do you want to watch from the sidelines? Do you want to take up a new exercise or hobby in your forties, fifties, and sixties or do you want to constantly say, 'That's not for me'? Do you want to still enjoy mobility when you are in your seventies and eighties, or do you want to be someone who can barely stand up from a chair because they haven't done any exercise in the previous decades? If all the answers are the first ones, then let's start working on it now.

MULTITASKING

We're all busy. We're all trying to juggle too much. We often know that we need to incorporate more exercise into our routine and, because we feel guilty, we begin a new programme or regime. We may start it with the best of intentions, but it often slips away within a few weeks. It isn't sustainable because it doesn't fit into our lives.

Instead of trying to carve out time from an already packed schedule, we need to build on what we already have. There are so many tasks we do within the day where we could be doubling up with a few quick exercises. Or there may be times when we have a couple of minutes while we are on the phone or lying in bed when we can stretch out our tired muscles. If we are low on free time, we should double up on the time we are already using.

> "IT ISN'T SUSTAINABLE BECAUSE IT DOESN'T FIT INTO OUR LIVES."

We want to form habits so that we find ourselves stretching our wrists or neck muscles without even thinking about it. Ideally, we want to be stretching every half an hour and standing up and moving around every hour. It doesn't need to be for a long time, just a couple of minutes. It's the consistency that's important and I've designed the following routines to target the areas of your body that most need help, depending on what activities you do during the day.

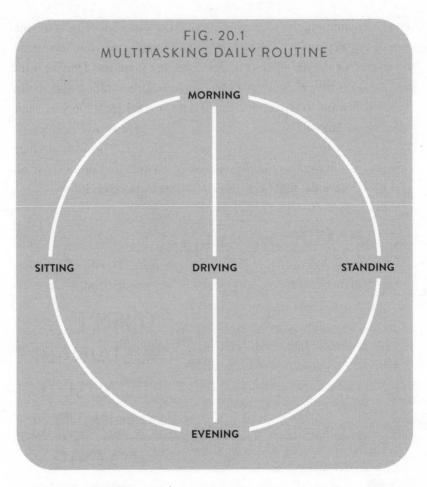

FIG. 20.1
MULTITASKING DAILY ROUTINE

MORNING

SITTING   DRIVING   STANDING

EVENING

I am going to start off in the morning with two routines designed around how you begin your day, then branch off into whether you mostly sit, stand, or drive during the day, and then we can meet back together in the evening on the couch (see Figure 20.1).

MORNING ROUTINE (IN BED)

Some people have a few minutes when they first wake up before they have to get out of bed. If you are one of these people, then use this time to gently stretch your body. Treat your bed like a yoga mat and try a new way to begin your day. It will awaken your body and mind before you even have to place your feet on the floor.

FIG. 20.2
BREATHING EXERCISE

FIG. 20.3
SELF-MASSAGE FOR
FRONT OF THE NECK

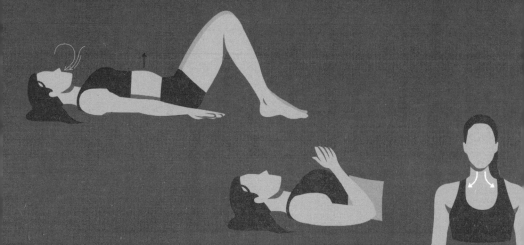

1

Raise your knees up so that your feet are flat on the mattress and your arms are straight down by your sides (see Figure 20.2). This is a good position to start with as it takes the pressure off your lower back. Start with a deep breath in through your nose, expanding your diaphragm. While breathing in try and push your belly button up to the ceiling. Slowly breathe out through your mouth, expelling all the air in your lungs. Gently return your breathing back to normal while consciously trying to breathe by raising your stomach rather than your chest.

2

Take both of your hands and place them under your chin, while leaving your knees in the same position. Use your finger pads to draw long, sweeping massage strokes down to your collarbone on both sides (see Figure 20.3). This will help loosen the muscles in the front of your neck that so often become tight with stress. Do this ten times.

FIG. 20.4
RESET FOR PELVIS
AND HIPS

FIG. 20.5
EXERCISE TO REDUCE
TIGHTNESS IN LEGS,
KNEES AND HIPS

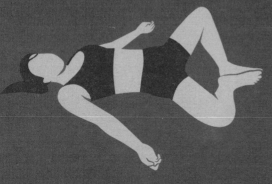

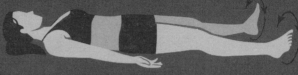

3

Place your hands by your sides again, but this time with the palms facing upwards (see Figure 20.4). With each of your knees angled to the side, bring the soles of your feet together so that your legs form a diamond shape. Hold this for twenty seconds. It will help reset the pelvis, open the hips, and take pressure off your lower back.

4

Straighten out your legs so your ankles are hip-width apart. Place your hands onto your stomach and leave them there, checking that you are still breathing by raising your stomach rather than your chest (see Figure 20.5). With your legs still straight, start rocking your toes inwards and outwards for two minutes. This will help lessen any stiffness or tightness in the legs, knees, and hips.

FIG. 20.6
ANKLE PUMPS

FIG. 20.7
GLUTE BRIDGES

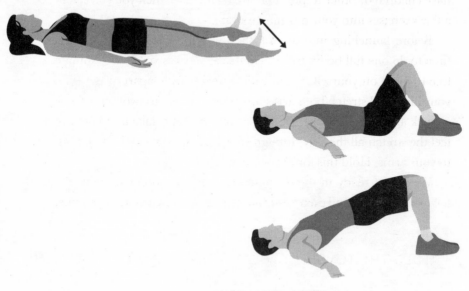

5

Point your toes down towards the wall and then up towards the ceiling (see Figure 20.6). Repeat this ten times. This is good for mobilization of the ankles and circulation, by bringing the blood back to your heart.

6

Finish off by raising your heartbeat slightly with some glute bridges. Bring your knees back up so that your feet are flat on the mattress and a hip-width apart. Place your arms so they are palms down and by your side. Gently use your legs to raise your hips away from the mattress (see Figure 20.7). Hold this position for three seconds and repeat this ten times. It will help strengthen your buttocks and the muscles in the back of your thighs. It's also good for your core strength.

You can now decide if you want to continue with the following, slightly more energetic routine for people who have to immediately get out of bed.

MORNING ROUTINE (OUT OF BED)

If you are someone who has to be out of bed straightaway because you have children or other responsibilities to attend to, then you can still fit a few exercises into your morning routine.

Before launching into any of the following exercises, take some time to do one full body stretch. Do this as soon as you have a minute free to focus on yourself. Stand with your feet wide apart (wider than your hips) and stretch both arms up and in the 'ten to two' position of a clock and lean back slightly. Close your eyes and take a moment to feel the stretch all the way through your legs, up to your chest and out to your arms. Hold this for thirty seconds.

We all get ready in the morning in a different order so move the following stretches and exercises around to suit your own morning routine:

FIG. 20.8
HOLD THE TOWEL IN THE 'TEN TO TWO' POSITION

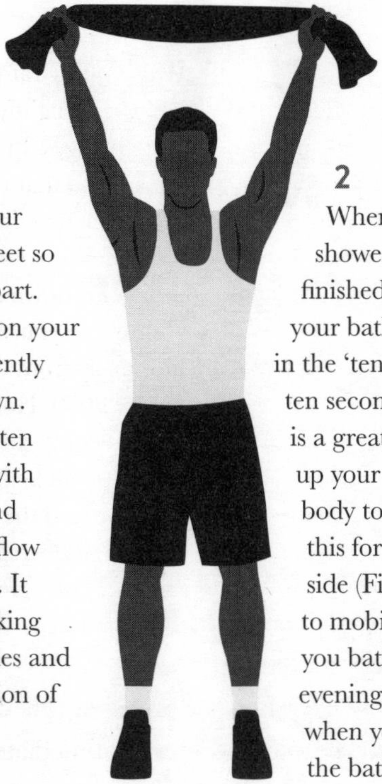

1

When brushing your teeth, move your feet so they are slightly apart. Raise yourself up on your tiptoes and then gently lower yourself down. Repeat this five to ten times. This helps with your circulation and encourages blood flow back to your heart. It also helps with waking up tight calf muscles and with the mobilization of the ankle.

2

When you get out of the shower or bath, and have finished drying yourself, hold your bath towel in your hands in the 'ten to two' position for ten seconds (Figure 20.8). This is a great exercise for opening up your chest. Next tilt your body to the side and hold this for ten seconds on each side (Figure 20.9). This helps to mobilize your back. If you bathe or shower in the evening, then do this exercise when you are getting ready in the bathroom in the morning.

FIG. 20.9
TILT YOUR BODY TO THE SIDE

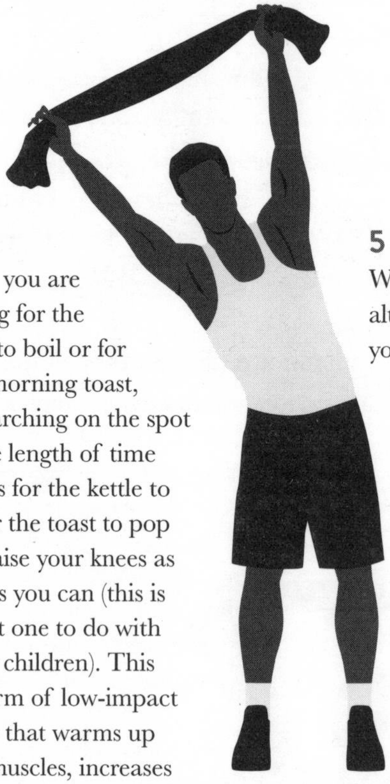

4

When you are waiting for the kettle to boil or for your morning toast, try marching on the spot for the length of time it takes for the kettle to boil or the toast to pop up. Raise your knees as high as you can (this is a great one to do with young children). This is a form of low-impact cardio that warms up your muscles, increases your heart rate, and improves circulation.

5

When you are getting dressed, alternate every item of nightwear you take off and clothing you put on with a deep squat. Do this with your feet wide and arms out to the side. Try and go as low as you feel comfortable with. Deep squats will help strengthen your buttocks and thigh muscles. It also helps the range of motion in your lower back, hips, knees, and ankles, will aid lower-back and pelvic stability, and will improve your posture. (There's a reason why exercise gurus love squats).

SITTING

If you find yourself sitting down for most of your day, there are lots of exercises you can do to counteract this position. Nearly all of them are subtle enough to do in even the busiest of office environments. We should try and do these exercises and stand up to move around for a minute or two every thirty minutes or every hour throughout the day.

FIG. 20.10
FIGURE-OF-EIGHT
NECK EXERCISE

FIG. 20.11
STRETCHES FOR WRISTS,
FOREARMS, AND BACK

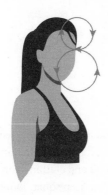

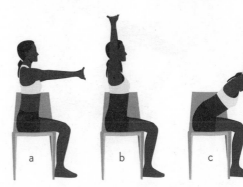

1

One of the best exercises for our neck is the 'figure of eight'. It sounds a bit odd, but imagine there are two pencils where your eyes are and draw a figure of eight with them (see Figure 20.10). Do this a few times, in both directions, and then imagine the pencils are where your nose is and do the same thing. Lastly place your imaginary pencils on your chin with it slightly raised and do a few more figures of eight in both directions. This helps mobilize the joints and stretches the muscles in your neck.

2

The following is a stretch for your wrists, forearms, spine, and the muscles linked to the mid and lower back. Interlace your fingers in front of you and push your arms out and away from your chest for ten seconds (Figure 20.11a). Raise your arms above your head and interlace your fingers, hold for ten seconds (Figure 20.11b). Sit on the edge of your chair and stretch your arms out in front of you at an angle and interlace your fingers (Figure 20.11c). Again, hold this for ten seconds. Finally, tilt your torso to the side and hold for ten seconds on each side.

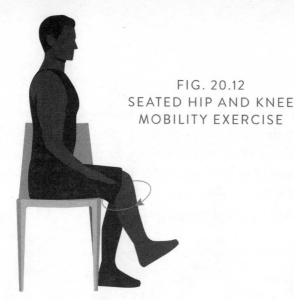

FIG. 20.12
SEATED HIP AND KNEE
MOBILITY EXERCISE

3

While sitting, raise one of your knees and keep your lower leg loose. Gently circle your knee both clockwise and anticlockwise five times (Figure 20.12). Do the same with your other leg. This movement is good for mobility in the hip and the knee. At the same time, if you want, you can add some ankle circles, five times clockwise and anticlockwise. This helps with the flexibility of the ankle.

4

When seated, and with your feet slightly apart, raise your calves as if you were standing on your tiptoes. Repeat this ten times. This helps with circulation, preventing swelling in the lower leg and ankle, and strengthens the calf muscles.

5

Stretch out your wrists to keep them mobile and help prevent any repetitive strain injuries. Hold your arms out in front of you and let your hand drop towards the floor. With your other hand, gently pull your wrist towards your body. Next, extend your wrist so your fingers are pointing up towards the ceiling and with your other hand, gently pull your fingers back towards your body. Hold both stretches for twenty seconds each and then repeat on your other wrist.

6

When you stand up to move around for a few minutes, you should firstly give each of your legs a shake as it will help with your circulation. If you're working from home, or if you are in an office and feel comfortable doing it, stand on one leg and pull your knee up to your chest and hold for a few seconds and repeat this on the other side. You can even do a few lunges if you want to incorporate these into your routine.

DRIVING

When it comes to driving, it is very important to do a few stretches before you get into the car. I always do this before a long drive and you will catch me doing a few extra stretches at the petrol station and service station as well. You are limited with what you can safely do inside the car so treat it as a pre-exercise warm-up instead.

Before you spend a long time in your vehicle you should:

FIG. 20.13
STRETCH FOR QUADS

FIG. 20.14
STRETCH FOR CALVES

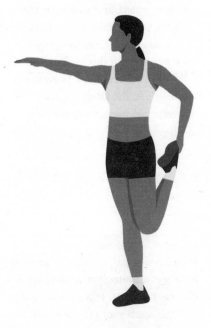

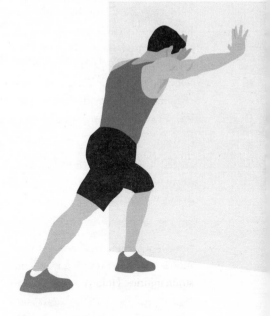

1

Stretch your quads out by pulling the heel of your foot up towards your bum (Figure 20.13). Hold this for ten seconds on each side.

2

Place both hands against a wall (or even your car) and stretch out your calf muscles and muscles in your chest by placing one leg further back than the other (Figure 20.14). Hold this for ten seconds on each side.

FIG. 20.15
LEG SWINGS

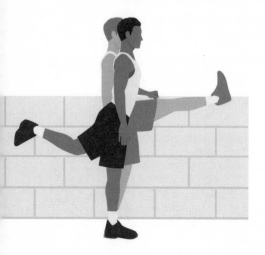

3

While standing, place one of your hands on a wall and gently swing your leg backwards and forwards five times. Turn to face the wall and swing the same leg from side to side five times. Do this with your other leg as well. This exercise helps with mobility in your hip.

When I am driving I have a small, hard ball, such as a baseball, lacrosse ball, or softball (which is my favourite) between my back and the car seat. This can be placed on the upper, middle, or lower back, the buttocks, or even the top of the hamstrings. The ball will press gently on the muscles when you are driving and help alleviate any tightness. It can also help support an upright posture when driving. You can either use two balls on either side of your spine or just one.

When you are stopped at a red light you can do the following stretches:

1

Place both hands behind your head and interlock your fingers. Pull your shoulder blades together (Figure 20.16). Hold for five to ten seconds. This helps stretch the muscles in your chest.

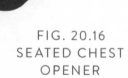

FIG. 20.16
SEATED CHEST
OPENER

FIG. 20.17
SEATED NECK SIDE
STRETCH

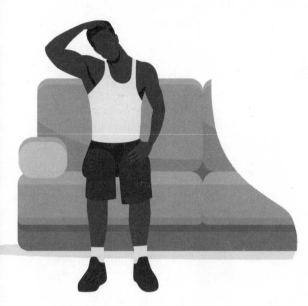

2

Tilt you right ear towards your right shoulder. Use your right hand to gently pull your head slightly closer to the shoulder (Figure 20.17). Hold for five to ten seconds. Do the same on the other side. Tilt your neck towards your chest and place both hands on the back of your head. Gently push your chin slightly closer to your chest. Hold for five to ten seconds. Both these exercises will help stretch out the muscles in the neck.

3

Hold your hands out in front of you and interlace your fingers so the palms are facing outwards. Drop your chin towards your chest. Hold for five to ten seconds. This stretches out the muscles in your back, arms, and shoulders.

STANDING

If your job requires you to stand all day, there are different exercises you can do to help the circulation in your legs. You should try and do these exercises every thirty minutes or every hour if you can.

FIG. 20.18
STANDING HEEL KICKS
TO HAND

FIG. 20.19
STANDING LEG
ABDUCTION

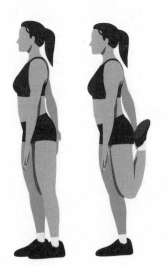

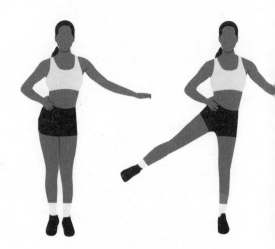

1

Place your hands at the base of your spine. Move one of your heels towards your hand before returning it to the ground and doing the same on the other side (Figure 20.18). Repeat this ten times. This helps increase the blood flow to the muscles, while also strengthening the core, hamstrings, and glutes.

2

Place your hands on your hips or, if you need to, extend one arm for balance, and lift one leg sideways, away from your body (Figure 20.19). Do this ten times on each side. This will help strengthen the hip, buttock, and thigh muscles.

3

Standing straight with your arms by your sides, gently slide your hands down towards your knees. Do this ten times on each side. This helps increase mobility in the spine, while also stretching it along with the abdominal obliques, TFL, and muscles in the back.

4

While standing, lift one leg up towards your chest and interlink your fingers around your knee and pull it closer to your chest. Maintain a straight back and hold for ten seconds before repeating on the other leg. This improves balance and stability, while also stretching the muscles in the back and legs.

5

Place all your body weight on your toes and then gently rock back onto your heels, while keeping your back straight. Do this rocking motion ten times. This helps improve circulation. It also increases the mobility of your ankle while strengthening the lower leg muscles.

6

Place one foot a little bit in front of the other and pull the heel off the ground. Slightly bend your knees. Use your hip to turn the whole leg inwards and outwards. Do this for ten seconds and then do the same on the heel of the foot. Repeat on the other side. This helps prevent tightness in the hip and surrounding muscles.

EVENING

Most of us end up on or near a couch for an hour or so in the evening. When I watch TV at night, I sit on the floor with my back against the sofa and my legs wide apart in front of me and alternate this with sitting cross-legged. This is better for your spine than curling up on a soft couch. It is also a great time to use a massage gun or foam roller. You can also try the following exercises:

1

While sitting on the edge of the sofa, hold your arms out in front of you and stand up. Do this a minimum of ten times and slowly build up to more. This will help strengthen your lower back and pelvis, while also being good for the flexibility of the lower back, hips, knees, and ankles.

FIG. 20.20
HIP STRENGTHENING EXERCISE ON SIDE

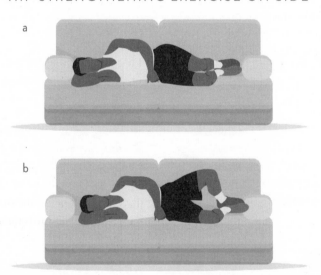

2

Lie on your side on the sofa with your arm bent and supporting the weight of your head (Figure 20.20a). Bend you knees slightly and then slowly raise the top leg, while keeping your feet together before lowering it back down (Figure 20.20b). Do this ten to fifteen times before repeating on the other side. This will strengthen the hips by working on the glutes. It can also help stabilize the pelvis and prevent lower-back and hip pain.

FIG. 20.21
DECOMPRESS YOUR LOWER BACK

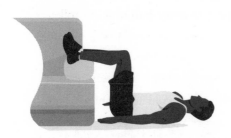

FIG. 20.22
HAMSTRING STRETCH ON CHAIR OR SOFA

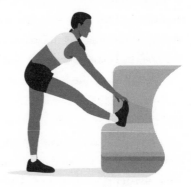

3

Lie on the ground and place your legs up on a sofa or chair so they are at a 90-degree angle (Figure 20.21). Hold this position for one to five minutes. This will help decompress the lower back while also assisting with realigning the lower back and pelvis. It also helps take away the tension from the facet joints and discs in the spine.

4

Place one leg on the couch and point your toes upwards. Keeping the leg straight, lean over and reach for your toes (Figure 20.22). Hold this for five seconds and repeat on the other leg. This alleviates tightness in the lower back and hamstring, as well as stretching out the calf.

FIG. 20.23
HIP FLEXOR STRETCH ON SOFA

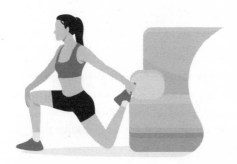

5

Drop into the lunge position (see Figure 20.23), making sure that the bent knee at the front is at an angle outwards rather than straight ahead and the knee behind is bent upwards and resting against the couch. You can place a pillow underneath your knee if it is sore as this will alleviate any pressure on it. Hold this position for ten seconds before repeating on the other side. This will stretch the psoas muscle in your lower back and your quads.

CARDIO

As well as stretches and exercises throughout the day, we also need a small amount of cardio to raise our heartbeats. Cardio is very important as it gets our circulation moving and helps regulate the different systems. It increases our metabolism, which means that we burn more calories, and it's also a great mood booster.

Cardio only needs to be done for twenty minutes a day, but the sessions can be combined to form longer ones. Ideally, it's better to do a little bit every day. I would recommend twenty minutes a day if you are doing the above stretches and exercises, but if you only have five minutes, make them count. Try and get your heart rate high in those five minutes. It's better to do something rather than nothing – even if it's just a short walk around the garden.

"IF WE DON'T INCLUDE CARDIO IN OUR LIVES THEN OUR FITNESS LEVELS DROP."

Our bodies need to be tested and if we don't include regular small amounts of cardio in our lives then our fitness levels quickly drop. This happens to everyone. The finest athletes in our country see a decrease of fitness when they train less, but this quickly returns if they take up their former routine. It's therefore important to keep your exercise consistent rather than doing an intense month and then having a month off.

Sometimes it's difficult to stick to twenty minutes of cardio a day, but often this is because we aren't enjoying what we are doing. We therefore need to think outside of the box when it comes to exercise. It doesn't have to be the traditional forms of going to the gym, running, or swimming. We can do team sports, or a brisk walk outside or on a treadmill. We can dance around the living room, climb up and down the stairs in our house, or find an app that gives us a different set of exercises each day. We can join a martial arts class or do some energetic cleaning or gardening. Try different things, set a timer, see which form of exercise goes by the quickest for you.

There may have been a time when you discovered a form of exercise that you enjoyed. It might have even been years ago, and your circumstances have now changed. You might have gone to a salsa class ten years ago, but can't do it now as you have three children. Try and adapt that exercise to your current lifestyle. Look for some pre-recorded salsa classes on the internet that you could access in the evenings, or when your children are at school. The key is to find something you enjoy and adapt it to your lifestyle. Make it fit with you, rather than bending to accommodate something that you won't want to continue with.

RECOVERY

Recovery time after exercising is important as it gives the body time to rest and repair. Sometimes, when we start a new exercise routine, we can suffer from aching muscles a day later. This is completely normal and means that there are tiny tears in our muscles that are healing. This is called Delayed Onset Muscle Soreness (DOMS) and will normally last between twenty-four and seventy-two hours. You will know that it is DOMS, rather than an injury, because it won't start until the day after exercising. There are a few things that can help with DOMS:

ICE MASSAGE

Straight after exercise, you can give yourself a relaxing massage by freezing water in a paper cup. Apply the ice on the sore spots around your body. You can then peel away the paper cup as the ice melts on your skin. I used to do this for the athletes I worked with during the Olympics and took this over to my private practice as well.

CONTRAST BATHING

As well as being good for aiding circulation, contrast bathing is also therapeutic. It helps with swelling, stiff joints, and pain relief. The theory behind it is that the heat expands the blood vessels and the cold constricts them, which helps with the blood-pumping mechanism. An easy way to do this is to switch between a hot towel and a cold one, or a hot shower followed by a cold one. If you are treating your feet, then you can put them into a cold basin and then a warm one – this is particularly good for people with Type 2 diabetes who have problems in their feet.

EPSOM SALT BATHS

Epsom salts contain magnesium and I find that these baths help relax my muscles. There is not much evidence supporting whether magnesium is absorbed through the skin, but I find them beneficial, even if they are a placebo. Advocates for Epsom salt baths say that they help reduce aching muscles, improve sleep, aid concentration, increase energy, and reduce inflammation in sore muscles.

If you think you might have injured yourself during exercise, then use your pain scale and **STOP** to assess the injury. If, when exercising, you experience stabbing or throbbing pains that are getting worse, then you should stop exercising straightaway.

If you have injured an area then, in most cases, you won't be helping your body by retreating to the couch and not moving for the next week. Instead, if you've injured the top half of your body then exercise the bottom half, and vice versa.

When returning to exercise after an injury, make sure you spend enough time warming up. This will also give you a chance to assess how your body is feeling and if the pain is returning. Start with walking drills, which might be walking slowly while lifting your knees high up. If that doesn't hurt, then continue with this for a couple of days before increasing your activity. The key is to build up to the exercise you were doing previously, rather than resting for a period and launching yourself straight back into it.

CHAPTER 21

Monthly Overhaul Treatment

(MOT)

To remain in the best condition, we need to spend some time every month releasing all the tension held in our body. This is a gift to ourselves. It is a time when we give ourself permission to do something relaxing and enjoyable, which also benefits our body.

A Monthly Overhaul Treatment (MOT) is a time to reset your body and reward yourself. We might have a massage once a year on holiday, by why leave it at that? Maybe you cannot afford to and, if that's the case, I've devised an introduction to all the skills you'll need to ease the strains on your body from the previous month. If you can afford a treatment every month then consider seeing a massage therapist, osteopath, or chiropractor for a restorative session. They can help reset your body, and you could even alternate this with going to a spa and using the sauna and ice bath there.

MASSAGE GUNS

In recent years, massage guns have become very popular. This is partly because you can use them by yourself on most areas of your body. They have also become very portable. Six years ago, I had a wired one that was so heavy that I felt like I needed a treatment every time I

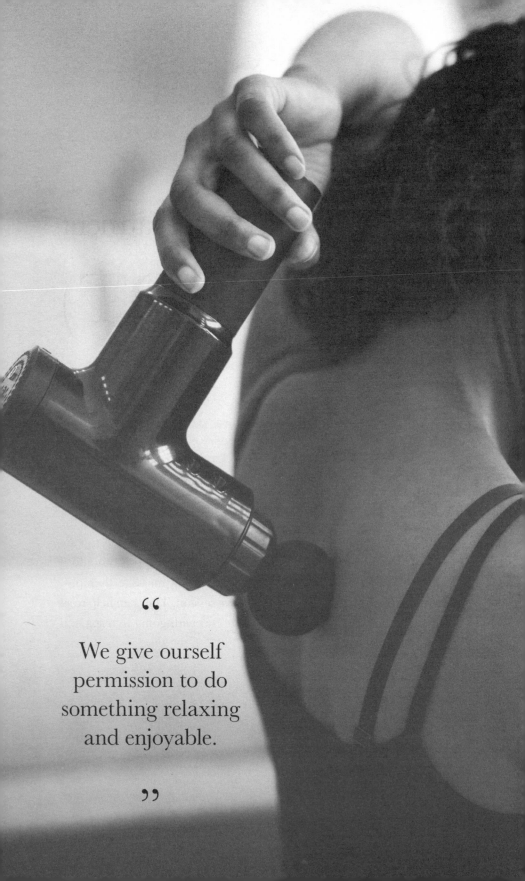

"
We give ourself
permission to do
something relaxing
and enjoyable.

"

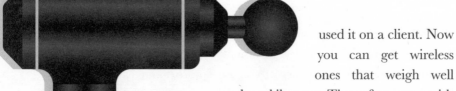

used it on a client. Now you can get wireless ones that weigh well under a kilogram. They often come with a small carry case that you can take wherever you are exercising. Their cost varies widely, but if you are going to be using it a lot, then you should invest in a more expensive massage gun as the cheaper ones tend to break. The expensive ones are also quieter.

They usually come with several interchangeable attachments that vibrate at a high frequency. You should only use the massage gun on an area for a maximum of one to two minutes, but you can come back to the same area later. You can either use it on yourself or ask a friend or family member to help.

THE BENEFITS OF A MASSAGE GUN	POINTS TO REMEMBER
• Reduces muscle soreness and stiffness	• Don't use a massage gun directly on a bone
• Prepares your body for a workout by improving the circulation	• Don't use it over bruises, cuts, or open wounds
• Can be used anywhere and anytime	• Never use it over an area that has a fracture
• Is an instant release for tired muscles	• Limit the time on an area to a maximum of two minutes. You can come back to an area later
• Can save you money as you won't need to see a therapist as much	

Massage guns normally come with four attachments, sometimes more (see Figure 21.1). The attachments with a larger surface area provide a more general massage. If you use a more pointed attachment, then the vibration is concentrated through a smaller surface area and will go deeper.

FIG. 21.1
MASSAGE GUN ATTACHMENTS

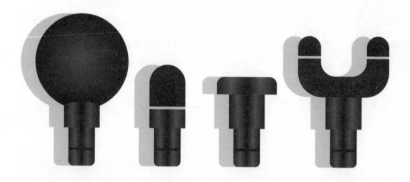

The ball attachment is the one that my clients seem to use the most as it's a midway attachment. It's used to treat large muscle groups in the body, such as the glutes, hamstrings, and quads. It covers a large area of the muscles as it can more easily treat the sides.

The bullet head is useful when targeting a specific area of muscle where you feel a tightness. For example, if you have tennis elbow, it can be directed onto the tendon just below the bony part of the elbow.

The flat head is the attachment that I use the most. Compared to the others, it's the best all-rounder that you can use on the main area of the muscles, from the chest through to the glutes, thighs, and legs. It works well between the shoulder blades as long as you don't use it over the bone or smaller muscles.

The forked attachment is used for both sides of the spine or the Achilles tendon. It can massage the muscles on either side of the spine without travelling over the bone.

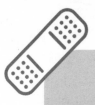

HOW TO USE A MASSAGE GUN

ON THE FRONT OF THE THIGH

- You can either be sitting or standing

- Place the massage gun on the front of the thigh and move it up and down

- Make sure you massage the outsides of the thigh muscles as well

- If you find a spot that is tender, hold the massage gun on it for twenty to thirty seconds

LOWER LEG

- Do this sitting down

- Place the massage gun on the back of the lower leg

- When massaging the front of the leg, shield the shin bone with your hand

- Make sure you cover the sides of the muscles as well

GLUTES

- You can do this either sitting, standing, or lying on your side

- Use the massage gun on all parts of the muscle

BACK OF THE THIGH

- You can either be standing or kneeling down

- Place the massage gun on your hamstrings, which are the large muscles at the back of the thigh

- Make sure you massage the inside, middle, and outsides of the muscles

LOWER BACK

- You can do this either sitting, standing, or lying down

- Only use the massage gun on the muscles to the sides of your spine and never directly on it

- The fork head is ideal for this area

SOLES OF THE FEET

- Do this sitting down

- Run the ball attachment up and down the soles of the feet

MASSAGE BALLS

Using a small, hard ball such as a tennis ball, lacrosse ball, softball, or baseball is a cheaper alternative to a massage gun. I've tested all these balls and the best one is a softball as it's the perfect size. This is something you can do by yourself to target areas of muscle that are tight. You need to place the ball between yourself and either a wall or the floor. When you roll the ball around an area of your body you should try to notice any tender areas. If you find somewhere that is tender, then you should concentrate on moving the ball around there with as much pressure as you can tolerate for ten seconds, to see if the muscle will release. Then move on to another area before returning to the earlier one to check if it is still tight.

The best areas to use a massage ball are:

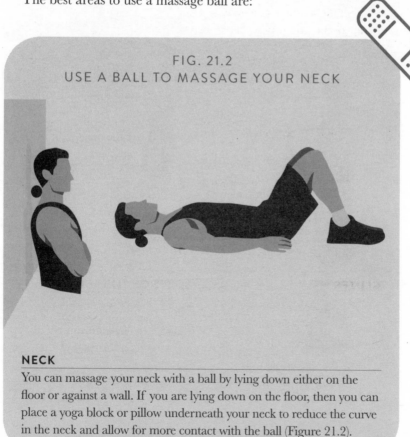

FIG. 21.2
USE A BALL TO MASSAGE YOUR NECK

NECK

You can massage your neck with a ball by lying down either on the floor or against a wall. If you are lying down on the floor, then you can place a yoga block or pillow underneath your neck to reduce the curve in the neck and allow for more contact with the ball (Figure 21.2).

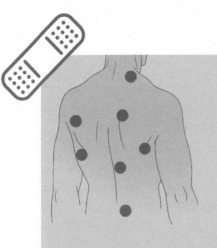

BACK

The illustration shows the areas to target on the back, depending on what exercise you have been doing (see Figure 21.3). If you are massaging around the shoulders, then pull your arms forward to allow maximum contact between the ball and the muscle (see Figure 21.4).

FIG. 21.3
WHERE TO PUT THE BALL TO MASSAGE YOUR BACK

FIG. 21.4
USE BALL TO MASSAGE SHOULDER

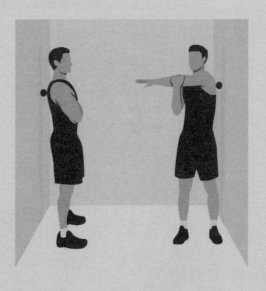

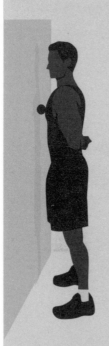

FIG. 21.5
HOW TO MASSAGE THE CHEST

CHEST

Our chest and the front of our shoulders are often neglected. The easiest way to massage these is against a wall, rather than on the floor (Figure 21.5).

FIG. 21.6
HOW TO MASSAGE GLUTES

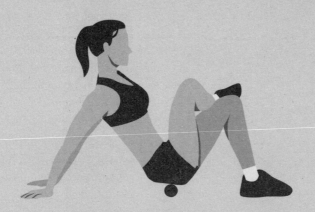

GLUTES

When massaging the glutes, either lying or sitting down, you can increase the pressure between the muscle and the ball by raising your leg and crossing it over the other one (Figure 21.6).

FIG. 21.7
HOW TO MASSAGE TIGHT HAMSTRINGS

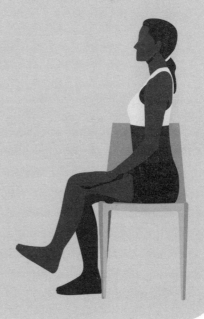

HAMSTRINGS

It's easiest to massage tight hamstrings if you can sit on a table and let your legs hang down (Figure 21.7). The weight of the leg naturally adds to the pressure on the muscle.

FIG. 21.8
HOW TO ALLEVIATE
TIGHT ARCHES AND
PLANTAR FASCIITIS

FEET

A massage ball can really
help with tight arches and
help alleviate plantar fasciitis
(Figure 21.8). You can do this
either standing or sitting.

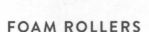

FOAM ROLLERS

Foam rollers are another cheaper option than a massage gun. I recommend them to clients when a muscle feels tight. You can also use them before, during, and after exercise. It's a quick, effective way of releasing a muscle and once you've bought a foam roller, they last for years. Because there is an element of balance to using a foam roller, they are also good for strengthening your core muscles.

There are several different ways that you can use a foam roller, but the following are three of my favourites that should each be done for two minutes at a time.

FIG. 21.9
RELEASING YOUR GLUTE MUSCLES

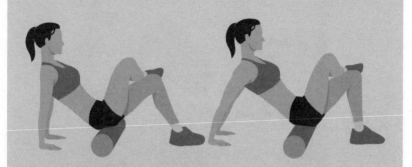

GLUTES

Sit on the foam roller at an angle to allow maximum contact between the muscles and the roller (Figure 21.9). Use a hand behind you for stability and move the roller by bending and straightening your knee.

FIG. 21.10
RELEASING YOUR THIGH MUSCLES

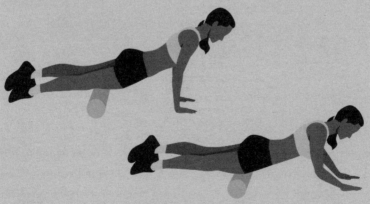

QUADS

Face the floor and place the foam roller between your thighs and the floor. Put your hands on the floor in a press-up position and let them take your weight. Use your arms to push the roller forwards and backwards (Figure 21.10). You can use the roller on both thighs at the same time or on each in turn.

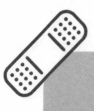

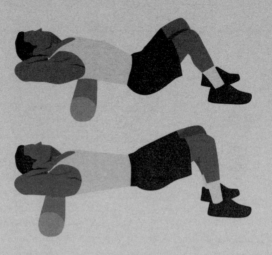

FIG 21.11
RELEASING YOUR BACK MUSCLES

BACK

Lie down on the foam roller with it placed at the top of your back. Interlink your fingers behind your head to support your neck (Figure 21.11). Bend and straighten your knees to move the roller across your back. You might feel a click in your spine, but if you do it's nothing to worry about. After you have done this for two minutes, move the foam roller further down to your lower back and repeat.

ASSISTED STRETCHES

Assisted stretches are something that you can do with a family member or friend, and you can take it in turns to help each other. Assisted stretches reinforce the stretches you do by yourself. Communication is key with assisted stretches. The person who is receiving them should let the other person know when they feel the stretch, and then the stretch should be held at that point for twenty seconds to prevent any of the muscles being overstretched.

Here are a few of my favourite assisted stretches:

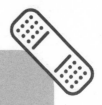

FIG. 21.12
ASSISTED GLUTE STRETCH

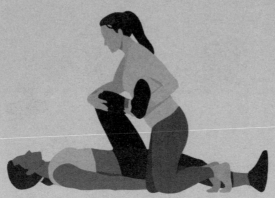

GLUTE STRETCH

Lie on your back and lift one leg up and bend it at the knee. The other person will then gently push your knee inwards and upwards in the direction of your shoulder (Figure 21.12). Repeat on the other leg.

FIG 21.13
ASSISTED HAMSTRING STRETCH

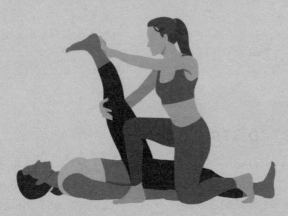

HAMSTRING STRETCHES

Lie down on the floor and raise your leg. The other person will place one hand on your foot and the other around your knee. They should then gently press the leg towards the chest (Figure 21.13). They should also loop their foot over your leg to prevent it from rising. Repeat on the other leg.

ADDUCTORS STRETCH FOR INNER THIGH

Lie down on the floor and raise both of your legs. The other person will then slowly push your legs apart to help stretch the muscles in your inner thigh (Figure 21.14).

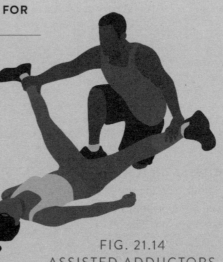

FIG. 21.14
ASSISTED ADDUCTORS
STRETCH

FIG. 21.15
ASSISTED HIP FLEXOR
STRETCH

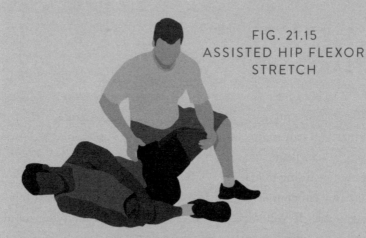

HIP FLEXOR STRETCH

Lie down on your side on either a bed or the floor. Bend both your knees and hold the knee that is closest to the floor with both hands. The other person positions themselves behind you and holds one foot with one hand and your knee with the other. They should then pull your leg gently behind you (Figure 21.15). The stretch is felt at the front of your thigh.

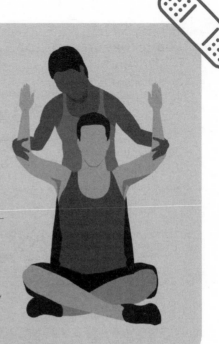

FIG. 21.16
ASSISTED CHEST
STRETCH

CHEST STRETCH

Sit down on the side of the bed
and lift up your arms. Keep your
head straight. The other person
should kneel behind you and pull
your arms backwards at the elbow
so you can feel a stretch across
your chest (Figure 21.16).

MASSAGE

Over the years, I have shown many clients simple massage techniques
that they can use on a partner or friend. There are so many different
ways that you can massage, and as you grow more confident in the
basics, you can begin to learn more techniques. It is an endless and
endlessly rewarding craft.

You can either massage each other on a bed or you can buy a
massage table. If you decide to massage on a bed, then you should
cover it with towels so that you don't get oil on the sheets. I have
tried many different types of oils, but I always come back to my two
favourites: shea butter and almond oil (this isn't suitable if you have a
nut allergy). I mix them together as they allow my hands to glide along
the muscles with the right amount of drag and pressure.

When massaging, your aim is to relax the muscles while also feeling
for any particularly tight areas or knots. Work on a tight muscle or
knot for ten seconds before moving on to another area, and then later

return to it if you need to. Use your body weight to apply the pressure rather than using the grip from your hands as this will prevent any strained muscles or tendons in your hands.

Here are a few massaging techniques to get you started.

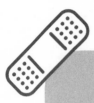

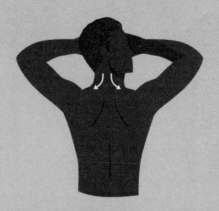

FIG. 21.17
MASSAGING THE NECK

NECK

Start off with the person lying on their front. Gently squeeze both sides of the shoulders. Run your thumbs up either side of the neck, all the way up to the base of the skull (Figure 21.17). Repeat this a few times until you feel the neck muscles begin to relax.

BACK OF THE LEGS

Place both your hands on the calf and push up the length of the leg to the top of the thigh. Pull back down again in one long, smooth motion. Repeat this for five minutes, adjusting the starting position so you cover all parts of the muscles.

ARMS

Ask the person to turn over so they are lying on their back. Start at the wrist and do circular movements up to the shoulder and back down again.

A Monthly Overhaul Treatment (MOT) is just as important as all the other suggestions and advice you have read. By either seeing a therapist or going through the above practices we can tease out all the stresses and strains we have added in the previous month and reset ourselves for the coming weeks. All of this will help reduce injuries, lower our stress levels, and leave us feeling more energized.

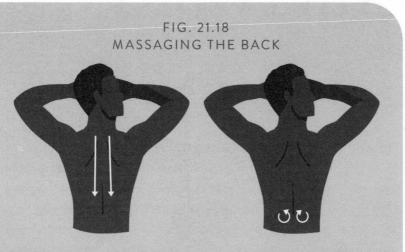

FIG. 21.18
MASSAGING THE BACK

BACK

Stand near the person's head and place both of your hands on either side of their spine, around their shoulders. Push both your hands slowly down the back and when you are lower down on the spine, use your thumbs to massage in circles on either side of the spine (Figure 21.18). Repeat this several times.

HANDS

Massage between the thumb and index finger. Next do small circles across the palms of the hands and along the fingers.

FRONT OF THE LEGS

Place both your hands on either side of their ankle. Glide your fingers all the way up to the hip and back down again. Start off in a slightly different place so that you cover all parts of the muscles.

FEET

Finish off with the feet. Concentrate on the soles and use both thumbs to do circular motions.

Afterword

The road map of STOP, SPACE, and MOT is a journey on which you can educate yourself about your body, find answers, and form realistic habits. By listening to the messages our bodies are sending us, we can learn to notice the warning signs and respond to them. We can then bring some balance into our lives and begin to reward ourselves.

It's important to have a strategy to combat pain, but it's better to have a strategy that can prevent it, and with SPACE and MOT you will be able to do this. Seeing a therapist for treatment is just one piece of the pie. Make your own rules if you need to. I am not here to shame you into doing twenty minutes or an hour of cardio a day, but if we can commit to something that is realistic, fun, and sustainable, the rewards will come. We are each a unique individual with one body that has to last us a lifetime. What better time than now to make a change?

Take a look at the following resources if you want to read more about the topics we've discussed. I wish you all the best on your own journey to body freedom, and if you share it please use the hashtag #resetwithjd so that I can hear all about it.

Resources

The following list includes organizations that you can refer to in order to check whether your therapist is registered, as well as for more general information about treatments.

British Chiropody and Podiatry Association (www.bcha-uk.org)

Chartered Society of Physiotherapists (www.csp.org.uk)

Complementary and Natural Healthcare Council (www.cnhc.org.uk)

Federation of Holistic Therapists (www.fht.org.uk).

General Chiropractic Council (www.gcc-uk.org)

General Osteopathic Council (www.osteopathy.org.uk)

Health and Care Professions Council (www.hcpc-uk.org)

National Health Service (NHS) (www.nhs.uk)

National Institute for Health and Care Excellence (NICE) (nice.org.uk)

World Health Organization (WHO) (www.who.int)

About the Author

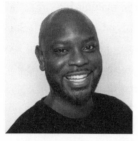

James Davies is a world-renowned osteopath, performance coach, and massage therapist. He has worked in the UK, USA, and Jamaica, with professional athletes ranging from Olympic champions and Premiership footballers to NFL and rugby union players, as well as with international A-list actors and musicians. As a performance therapist and athletics coach, James is able to integrate osteopathy, massage, acupuncture, biomechanics, and functional and structural applications. He is the founder and CEO of the Rising Health Osteopathy and Massage Clinic, and developed its ethos of 'relieve, restore, and perform', based on his own personal experience as a young athlete. James now works with people from all backgrounds.

Thankyous

Thank you to my parents for loving me, and for drilling into me the fundamentals of hard work. Thank you to my older brothers for being my role models, my guides, and my friends. Thank you to my wife for supporting me throughout my career and always remaining calm. Thank you to my kids for giving me purpose and laughter. Thanks also to:

Nik Raicevic for the love of sport.

The Olympics for the experience.

Sue Palfreyman, your three to four hour lessons every Friday at university made me fall in love with anatomy.

Kyle Sinckler for the belief and always being steadfast.

Anthony Watson for being kind and true.

Jonathan Joseph for the honesty.

Samuel Hill for Shinjuku, Tokyo.

Tez for the adventures.

Jay Anthony for your youthful spirit.

Dennis Elvie for the music.

Neil Kingston for being a good egg.

David Jason for the laughs.

Tim Swiel for the advice.

Tyrone Mings for being the first.

Deborah Reid for being an angel.

Linford Christie for the dream.

Dr Uchenna Okoye for Gloucester Road.

Tanser Shinasi, George Brobbey, and Jonathan Edosomwan, for the brotherhood.

Anthony Toumazou for your humanity.

Eamonn Holmes for the life lessons.

Tom Austen for the sight.

Greg Guillon my first flatmate, for the clarity.

James Dasaolu for the loyalty and ideas.

Ollie Thorley for the talks.

David Beckham for being my hero. The old saying – 'You should never meet your hero' – is completely wrong.

Mary Noble and Mandy Smith, for the English.

Perri (Shakes-Drayton) Edwards for being a superstar.

Charlotte Hills and Georgina Woolfrey for the band of joy.

Sarah Spendloff, Himesh Tailor, Michelle Blythe, Colin Houston, and Anne-Marie Houston, for the memories.

Nilam Holmes, the woman who never ages and is the hardest-working person I know. Thank you for opening the door.

Jane Dodd for helping me clear my mind and look ahead.

Patrick Morgan for the constant help and support.

Kylie Minogue for being a beautiful soul.

Joe Wicks for inspiring me and being my ice-bath buddy.

Marvin Humes and Rochelle Humes, for being you.

Michelle Campbell for being my sister from another mother.

Wendy Rowe for being spectacular always.

HarperCollins for giving me the opportunity to share my passion with the world.

Amy Warren for your sacrifice and many talents.

My agent, Bev James, for making this happen.

And to all my patients over the years – thank you for allowing me to help you.

Index

TFL muscle 233
therapists
 alternative and complementary
  312–315
 getting the best out of appointments
  284–285
 selection 282, 285–286, 315
thighs
 assisted stretch 404
 foam roller release 401
 referred pain 216, 224
thread the needle 151
tiredness 366–369
tissue repair
 non-invasive 302–306
 RICE treatment 71
TMJ disorder 97–99
Tok Sen 320–321
traction 31, 211
traction machines 117
training
 chronic pain case study 61
 healthy pain 49–51
 performance therapy 311
trapezius muscle 104, 107, 138, 300
trigeminal neuralgia 46, 100

U
ulcerative colitis 192
ultrasound 31, 303
'unhappy triad,' knees 252

V
vagus nerve 339–340
vertebrae fractures 55, 149
visceral organs 178, 192
visceral pain 37
voice box 117

W
walking 365–366
water intake 367
weight, connection to knee osteoarthritis
 256
weightlifting 142, 160, 210
work
 physical warm ups 55, 156
 shoulders 123
wrists

bones 167
carpal tunnel syndrome 172–175
ganglion cysts 176
massage 164, 174–175
repetitive strain injury (RSI) 176
STOP pain description 168–170,
 174
stretches and exercises 176–177
warning signs 168

Y
yoga
 child's pose 150, 221
 overview 31, 321
 thread the needle 151

Image credits

CHAPTER OPENERS

HQ

An imprint of HarperCollins*Publishers* Ltd
1 London Bridge Street
London SE1 9GF

www.harpercollins.co.uk

HarperCollins*Publishers*
Macken House, 39/40 Mayor Street Upper,
Dublin 1, D01 C9W8, Ireland

10 9 8 7 6 5 4 3

First published in Great Britain by
HQ, an imprint of HarperCollins*Publishers* Ltd 2022

HB ISBN 978-0-00-852406-7
TPB ISBN 978-0-00-852407-4

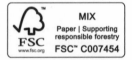

This book is produced from independently certified FSC™ paper
to ensure responsible forest management.

For more information visit: www.harpercollins.co.uk/green

Printed and Bound in the UK using 100% Renewable Electricity
at CPI Group (UK) Ltd, Croydon, CR0 4YY

Publishing Director: Rose Sandy
Editorial Assistant: Emily Kiel
Illustration: Charlotte Phillips
Designed by Kieron Lewis | KieronLewis.com
Page Design/Typesetting: e-Digitaldesign

All photographs © SHUTTERSTOCK
except author photograph: Barry Scowen